Management of Shock - Recent Advances

Edited by Amit Agrawal and Vaishali Waindeskar

Published in London, United Kingdom

Management of Shock - Recent Advances
http://dx.doi.org/10.5772/intechopen.100997
Edited by Amit Agrawal and Vaishali Waindeskar

Contributors
Naveed ur Rehman Siddiqui, Numair Belgaumi, Ahmed Salik, Franco Turani, Sara Martini, Samuel Jacob, Pankaj Garg, Saqib Masroor, Ishaq Wadiwala, John H. Yazji, Mohammad Alomari, Md Walid Akram Hussain, Emad Alamouti-Fard, Mohamed Samir Hassan Elawady, Amit Agrawal, Sri Rama Ananta Nagabhushanam Padala, Vaishali Waindeskar, Ved Prakash Maurya, Rakesh Mishra

First published in London, United Kingdom, 2023 by IntechOpen
IntechOpen is the global imprint of INTECHOPEN LIMITED, registered in England and Wales, registration number: 11086078, 5 Princes Gate Court, London, SW7 2QJ, United Kingdom

British Library Cataloguing-in-Publication Data
A catalogue record for this book is available from the British Library

Additional hard and PDF copies can be obtained from orders@intechopen.com

Management of Shock - Recent Advances
Edited by Amit Agrawal and Vaishali Waindeskar
p. cm.
Print ISBN 978-1-80356-314-5
Online ISBN 978-1-80356-315-2
eBook (PDF) ISBN 978-1-80356-316-9

Meet the editors

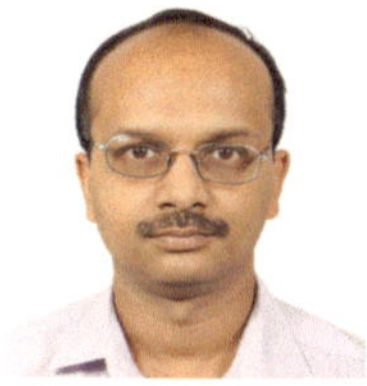

Dr. Agrawal completed his neurosurgery training at the National Institute of Mental Health and Neurosciences, Bangalore, India, and is now a member of many field-related societies including the World Federation of Neurological Societies, Congress of Neurological Societies, American Association of Neurological Surgeons, International Stroke Society, World Association of Medical Editors, Indian Society of Neuro-oncology, and World Endoscopic Spine Society.

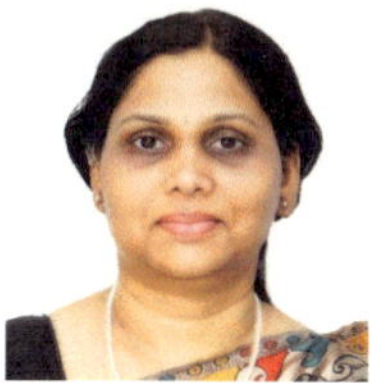

Dr. Waindeskar has vast experience in managing patients in anesthesia practice. She worked closely to develop the Anesthesia Department and critical care services at All India Institute of Medical Sciences, Bhopal, India. Her interests include pediatric anesthesia, pain and palliative care, intensive care, and ultrasound-guided block anesthesia procedures.

Contents

Preface

Shock is a clinico-pathologic state characterized by a mismatch between oxygen demand and oxygen delivery leading to tissue hypoxia and impairment of physiological functions. If the underlying precipitating factors are not identified, then the initial compensatory phase can be followed by a cascade of neuroendocrine compensatory mechanisms leading to decompensation and irreversible damage to organs and increased morbidity and mortality. Comprehensive management of a shock patient requires early diagnosis, identification of the underlying pathology, and a comprehensive goal-oriented management protocol. If left untreated or undetected, shock can result in life-threatening complications and negative outcomes. Hence, early detection should be the goal of physicians involved in the management of cases with potential shock of any etiology. Shock can be categorized as septic shock, anaphylactic shock, cardiogenic shock, hypovolemic shock, and neurogenic shock. The broader objective should focus on early detection of shock to identify the underlying etiology and the type of shock, as well as determine management strategies. This book enhances understanding of shock, including its pathophysiological and clinical characteristics, and can help health practitioners to identify shock and develop effective management approaches.

Amit Agrawal
Professor,
Department of Neurosurgery,
All India Institute of Medical Sciences,
Bhopal, India

Vaishali Waindeskar
Department of Anesthesia and Critical Care,
All India Institute of Medical Sciences,
Bhopal, India

Chapter 1

Introductory Chapter: Concomitant Traumatic Brain Injury and Haemorrhagic Shock

Sri Rama Ananta Nagabhushanam Padala, Vaishali Waindeskar, Ved Prakash Maurya, Rakesh Mishra and Amit Agrawal

1. Introduction

Younger people in developing countries are more frequently affected by head injuries, which have substantial economic and social effects. In patients with traumatic brain injury (TBI), external or internal haemorrhages have the potential to cause systemic hypotension [1, 2]. They can be associated with poorer outcomes (increased morbidity and mortality) compared to patients with TBI alone [3, 4]. Even brief episodes of hypotension have been shown to cause both systemic and cerebral hypoperfusion and secondary brain injury [5]. This systemic hypertension can be further complicated by raised intracranial pressure (due to TBI-related lesions), which can further compound the treatment protocols [6]. In trauma patients, the occurrence of haemorrhagic shock is associated with high mortality (as high as 50%) [7], and the reported incidence ranges from 6-16% [8]. These cases need to be differentiated from those in the paediatric population, where the isolated TBI can lead to severe shock (in the absence of apparent haemorrhage) [9, 10]. Understanding the interaction of the simultaneous presence of TBI and haemorrhagic shock is essential to implement the optimal resuscitation strategy [11] and, thus, developing strategies to improve outcomes in this subgroup of patients [5]. Investigators have used animal models to define the optimal post-resuscitation mean arterial pressure levels to ensure organ perfusion and, thus, maintain good organ functions and survival patterns [2]. The present article discusses the concepts and controversies associated with concurrent TBI and haemorrhagic shock, the clinical approach, and the management of this subgroup of patients.

2. Clinical examination

The clinical examination of a patient with suspected haemorrhagic shock and TBI is aimed at determining the source of the bleeding from any systemic external or internal injuries and understanding the severity of the head injury. The cursory examination of the neurological status involves the evaluation of the Glasgow Coma

Scale (GCS) and pupils, which will help assess the need for further radiological evaluation or urgent surgical intervention. One should be mindful that haemorrhagic shock is one of the confounding factors in the assessment of GCS. The detailed examination of the patient must include an assessment of the airway, breathing, circulation, and disability. While the patient is being stabilized, the neurological examination and examination to rule out other injuries like haemothorax, hemoperitoneum, or long bone fractures will continue, and appropriate measures can be taken to control the ongoing haemorrhage, if any. It is important to remember that the scalp can be a significant source of bleeding in children and should be scrutinized. In a patient with TBI and shock, bilaterally dilated and fixed pupils (in the absence of local injury and any drug overdose) can be an ominous sign that signifies a poorer outcome [12].

3. Diagnosis

Haemorrhagic shock in a patient with traumatic brain injury must be defined using a standard definition in the given setting [13, 14]. The diagnosis of traumatic brain injury and haemorrhagic shock will be evident in most cases. However, a careful clinical evaluation, including a detailed clinical history that can be supplemented with appropriate investigations, is needed to assess the extent of brain injury and haemorrhagic shock [14]. The detailed laboratory investigations shall include complete blood counts (including haemoglobin levels), a coagulation profile, and imaging of the brain or approximate regions to find the cause of haemorrhagic shock.

4. Management

Management of TBI with haemorrhagic shock remains a challenge [13] which is further compounded by the fact that there is wide variability in clinical practices. Various parameters must be kept in mind while managing this patient population, including intracranial pressure monitoring, a coagulation profile, an optimum blood pressure target, and the issue of performing combined surgical procedures for a combination of injuries [13]. In addition to the standard management protocol, the objective of management in these cases is "hemodynamic and haemostatic resuscitation" [13]. An optimal blood pressure management strategy will be necessary as there may be a combination of systemic hypotension and intracranial hypertension. It will be better to maintain the systemic blood pressure on the higher side [15]. The management strategy in these patients is debatable; however, the management should focus on the management of hypotension, cerebral oedema, coagulopathy (if present), judicious use of antiepileptics, and blood replacement [13]. As recommended, tranexamic acid can be given to reduce the mortality rate in these patients [16]. A few words of caution: aggressive fluid resuscitation in these patients must be avoided as it may have deleterious effects and increase short-term mortality [17]. Although head-end elevation is a standard practice in managing patients with TBI and raised intracranial pressure, its role in managing these patients is controversial [18]. Similarly, the role of the Trendelenburg position, which has been suggested to improve transient hypotension in haemorrhagic shock [19], is doubtful [20]. Maintain a neutral head and neck position to prevent jugular compression which would further impede venous return to the heart in the background of haemorrhagic shock.

5. Outcome

The outcome of patients who sustain TBI and concomitant haemorrhagic shock is unfavourable. It has been reported that 33-50% of patients die before they can reach the hospital [21]. These patients' significant causes of mortality are exsanguination and its sequelae, multi-organ dysfunction and coagulopathy [13]. Brain injury-related insults aggravate cardiovascular dysfunction and result in poorer outcomes [22]. TBI can cause cerebral oedema, requiring a higher systemic blood pressure to maintain cerebral perfusion. On the other hand, systemic hypotension in haemorrhagic shock results in decreased mean arterial pressure and subsequent decreased cerebral perfusion pressure. This interdependent impairment of haemodynamic regulatory mechanisms in a vicious cycle further leads to unfavourable outcomes [22].

6. Conclusions

In summary, patients with concomitant TBI and haemorrhagic shock usually sustain multisystem injuries that need an urgent and comprehensive team approach and may receive excellent pre-hospital care wherever possible. Although in most patients with TBI, shock is caused by haemorrhage, TBI can cause shock, particularly in the paediatric population. In either circumstance, the main objective is early identification of the underlying pathology and comprehensive management of responsible pathologies to improve outcomes. In traumatic intracranial pathologies, there may be a mismatch between systemic blood pressure and intracranial pressure that needs to be closely monitored to maintain optimal cerebral perfusion pressure.

Conflict of interest

The authors have NO conflict of interest to declare.

Author details

Sri Rama Ananta Nagabhushanam Padala[1], Vaishali Waindeskar[1], Ved Prakash Maurya[2], Rakesh Mishra[3] and Amit Agrawal[4*]

1 Department of Anesthesia and Critical Care, All India Institute of Medical Sciences, Bhopal, Madhya Pradesh, India

2 Department of Neurosurgery, Sanjay Gandhi Post Graduate Institute of Medical Sciences, Lucknow, India

3 Department of Neurosurgery, Institute of Medical Sciences, Trauma Centre and Mahamana Centenary Superspeciality Hospital, Banaras Hindu University, Varanasi, India

4 Department of Neurosurgery, All India Institute of Medical Sciences, Bhopal, Madhya Pradesh, India

*Address all correspondence to: dramitagrawal@gmail.com

References

[1] Gennarelli TA et al. Comparison of mortality, morbidity, and severity of 59,713 head injured patients with 114,447 patients with extracranial injuries. The Journal of Trauma. 1994;**37**(6):962-968

[2] Hu Y et al. Identification of ideal resuscitation pressure with concurrent traumatic brain injury in a rat model of hemorrhagic shock. The Journal of Surgical Research. 2015;**195**(1):284-293

[3] Matsushita Y et al. Delayed hemorrhagic hypotension exacerbates the hemodynamic and histopathologic consequences of traumatic brain injury in rats. Journal of Cerebral Blood Flow and Metabolism: Official Journal of the International Society of Cerebral Blood Flow and Metabolism. 2001;**21**(7):847-856

[4] Wald SL, Shackford SR, Fenwick J. The effect of secondary insults on mortality and long-term disability after severe head injury in a rural region without a trauma system. The Journal of Trauma. 1993;**34**(3):377-381

[5] Doyle JA, Davis DP, Hoyt DB. The use of hypertonic saline in the treatment of traumatic brain injury. The Journal of Trauma. 2001;**50**(2):367-383

[6] Hariri RJ et al. Traumatic brain injury, hemorrhagic shock, and fluid resuscitation: Effects on intracranial pressure and brain compliance. Journal of Neurosurgery. 1993;**79**(3):421-427

[7] Sauaia A et al. Epidemiology of trauma deaths: A reassessment. The Journal of Trauma. 1995;**38**(2):185-193

[8] Kauvar DS, Lefering R, Wade CE. Impact of hemorrhage on trauma outcome: An overview of epidemiology, clinical presentations, and therapeutic considerations. The Journal of Trauma. 2006;**60**(6 Suppl):S3-S11

[9] Gardner A et al. Isolated head injury is a cause of shock in pediatric trauma patients. Pediatric Emergency Care. 2013;**29**(8):879-883

[10] Partrick DA et al. Is hypotension a reliable indicator of blood loss from traumatic injury in children? American Journal of Surgery. 2002;**184**(6):555-559

[11] Investigators SS et al. Saline or albumin for fluid resuscitation in patients with traumatic brain injury. The New England Journal of Medicine. 2007;**357**(9):874-884

[12] Youmans JR. Causes of shock with head injury. Journal of Trauma and Acute Care Surgery. 1964;**4**(2):204-209

[13] Chico-Fernández M et al. Concomitant traumatic brain injury and hemorrhagic shock: Outcomes using the Spanish Trauma ICU Registry (RETRAUCI). The American Surgeon. 2021;**87**(3):370-375

[14] Galvagno SM et al. Outcomes after concomitant traumatic brain injury and hemorrhagic shock: A secondary analysis from the Pragmatic, Randomized Optimal Platelets and Plasma Ratios trial. The Journal of Trauma and Acute Care Surgery. 2017;**83**(4):668-674

[15] Spahn DR et al. The European guideline on management of major bleeding and coagulopathy following trauma: Fifth edition. Critical Care (London, England). 2019;**23**(1):98

[16] Collaborators, C.-T et al. Effects of tranexamic acid on death, vascular

occlusive events, and blood transfusion in trauma patients with significant haemorrhage (CRASH-2): A randomised, placebo-controlled trial. Lancet (London, England). 2010;**376**(9734):23-32

[17] Stern SA et al. Effect of initially limited resuscitation in a combined model of fluid-percussion brain injury and severe uncontrolled hemorrhagic shock. Journal of Neurosurgery. 2000;**93**(2):305-314

[18] Choi DS et al. Effects of position on intracranial pressure management in porcine traumatic brain injury with hemorrhagic shock. Emergency Medicine, Trauma and Surgical Care. 2021;**8**(1):1-7

[19] Martin JT. The Trendelenburg position: A review of current slants about head down tilt. AANA Journal. 1995;**63**(1):29-36

[20] Bridges N, Jarquin-Valdivia AA. Use of the Trendelenburg position as the resuscitation position: To T or not to T? American Journal of Critical Care: An Official Publication, American Association of Critical-Care Nurses. 2005;**14**(5):364-368

[21] Ling G et al. Explosive blast neurotrauma. Journal of Neurotrauma. 2009;**26**(6):815-825

[22] Yuan XQ, Wade CE. Traumatic brain injury attenuates the effectiveness of lactated Ringer's solution resuscitation of hemorrhagic shock in rats. Surgery, Gynecology & Obstetrics. 1992;**174**(4):305-312

Chapter 2

Shock Pathophysiology: Classifications and Management

Numair Belgaumi, Ahmed Salik
and Naveed ur Rehman Siddiqui

Abstract

Shock is a pathological state in which there is an insufficiency in oxygen supply and demand. Ultimately, it results in global hypoperfusion and a resulting increase in anaerobic respiration causing lactic acidosis. Maintaining adequate oxygen delivery in the critical care setting is of primary importance in the management of a critically ill patient. When oxygen supply is inadequate, the body undergoes several physiological changes to maintain the oxygen delivery requirements and perfusion pressure. This stage is referred to as compensated shock, and early signs of shock may be appreciated during this stage. When compensatory mechanisms are inadequate and DO_2 begins to fall beyond the critical point, shock has progressed to the uncompensated stage. During this stage, there is rapid deterioration of the patient due to prolonged hypoxia and anaerobic respiration. Multiple Organ Dysfunction Syndrome (MODS) is the development of potentially reversible physiological derangement involving two or more organ systems not involved in the causative disorder, which results in persisting states of shock, sepsis and hypoperfusion and a major cause of high mortality in the intensive care unit reaching a range of 11–54% in septic pediatric patients. The final stage of shock is irreversible shock, which is also referred to as refractory shock. This final stage of shock carries a 96–99% mortality rate.

Keywords: shock, hypovolemic shock, cardiogenic shock, distributive shock, obstructive shock, oxygen delivery, cardiac output, compensated shock, uncompensated shock, resuscitation, management, inotropes

1. Introduction

Shock is a pathological state in which there is an insufficiency in oxygen supply and demand. Ultimately it results in global hypoperfusion and a resulting increase in anaerobic respiration causing lactic acidosis. Adequate oxygen delivery is an essential requirement for the sustenance of every cell in the body, the lack of which can result from a variety of pathological disturbances and can lead to life-threatening alterations. Therefore, maintaining adequate oxygen delivery in the critical care setting is of primary importance in the management of a critically ill patient.

2. Physiological need for oxygen

The requirement for oxygen is as important as a cell's need for biochemical energy, without which no cellular or biochemical process can occur. Of the various biochemical mediums for energy, ATP is the most crucial due to the inherently high energy stored within the bonds between phosphate groups. Additionally, these bonds are readily and quickly broken to yield energy stored due to their unstable nature [1]. While ATP can be produced by processes such as glycolysis and the Krebs cycle, the amount produced by oxidative phosphorylation during the reactions within the electron transport chain, an oxygen-dependent mechanism, is vastly greater than that which the other two processes can produce. Anaerobic metabolism is an important means by which tissues can continue to produce ATP in oxygen deprived states; however it does not yield enough energy to support the functional requirements of most tissues. Therefore, the need for adequate oxygenation and delivery of oxygen to tissues across the body is essential for normal physiology.

3. Oxygen delivery

For proper oxygenation of tissues, oxygen delivery is essential and is achieved by circulation of oxygenated blood. To understand the mechanisms and factors that influence delivery one must first understand certain terms and their interconnected influence on oxygen delivery.

Firstly, the term **oxygen delivery (DO_2)** refers to the rate at which oxygen is delivered per unit time to cells, tissues and organs. **Oxygen consumption (VO_2)** subsequently is the rate at which oxygen is consumed per unit time by a cell, tissue or organ [1]. We'll begin by discussing oxygen delivery and the essential factors that influence delivery.

Oxygen delivery is dependent on two factors, **Cardiac output (CO)** and **arterial oxygen content (CaO_2)**. A change in one of these can decrease or increase the amount of global oxygen delivery. Physiologically, these factors are not independent and changes in one will be compensated with changes in the other to maintain adequate DO_2. These components of DO_2 can be expressed (Eq. 1) as:

$$DO_2 = CO \times CaO_2 \tag{1}$$

3.1 Arterial oxygen content

At any given time, blood leaving the left ventricle will be oxygenated to a certain degree expressed as the **arterial oxygen content (CaO_2)**. This term refers both to the amount of **hemoglobin saturated with oxygen (SaO_2)** and the amount of **oxygen dissolved in blood (PaO_2)**. Furthermore, since hemoglobin accounts for most of arterial oxygenation, the **concentration of hemoglobin in blood (Hgb)** is also an important determinant of CaO_2 (**Figure 1**).

These three factors determining arterial oxygen content can be mathematically represented by the following formula (Eq. 2):

$$CaO_2 = (Hbg \times 1.34 \times SaO_2) + (PaO_2 \times 0.003) \tag{2}$$

As can be appreciated from this equation (Eq. 2) hemoglobin concentration and saturation account for a vast majority of arterial oxygenation with dissolved oxygen only making a fraction of the total oxygen level.

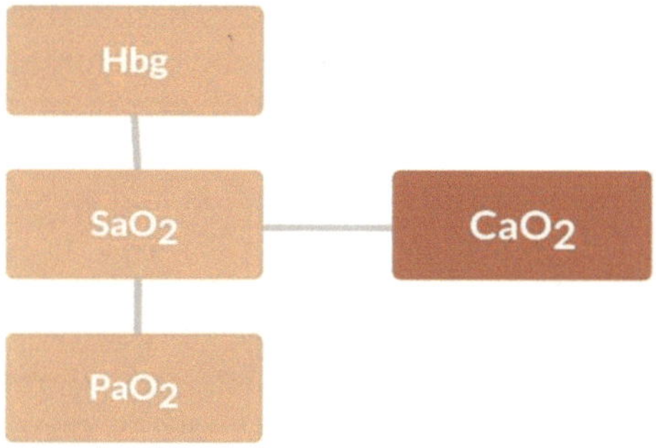

Figure 1.
Determinants of CaO_2.

3.2 Cardiac Output

Circulation of oxygenated blood allows for oxygen to reach the most distal parts of the body. Circulation is determined by the heart's functionality which is represented by cardiac output (CO). Factors that influence cardiac output are the **Stroke Volume (SV)** and the **Heart Rate (HR)**. The relationship of these measurements to cardiac output is expressed in the equation below (Eq. 3):

$$CO = SV \times HR \tag{3}$$

Stroke volume is defined as the amount of blood pumped from the left ventricle into the aorta within a single contraction. Three factors determine stroke volume: **Preload, Contractility,** and **Afterload**. These components are often difficult to directly assess clinically and are often estimated using indirect methods and assumptions. Preload refers to the amount of end-diastolic stress or pressure exerted on the walls of the left ventricle influencing myocardial sarcomere length. The major determinant of preload is venous pressure and subsequent venous return. Other factors influencing preload include ventricular wall compliance, atrial contractility and valvular resistance. End-diastolic volume is usually used as an estimate for preload. Contractility refers to the rate of sarcomere shortening during contraction. It represents the functionality of cardiac muscle and is influenced by stimulation via catecholamine and concentration of electrolytes such as calcium, magnesium and potassium. Afterload refers to the force against which the left ventricle contracts and is defined as the left ventricular wall stress.

4. Oxygen consumption and oxygen extraction

Oxygen consumption (VO_2) by cells and tissues is dependent on their energetic requirements and expenditure. It is defined as the amount of oxygen consumed per minute. The more metabolically active a tissue is the more oxygen it will require to maintain that activity. Therefore, oxygen consumption is a measure of energy expenditure. It can be expressed as the equation (Eq. 4) given below where $CmvO_2$ is the mixed venous oxygen content:

$$VO_2 = (CaO_2 - CmvO_2) \times CO \tag{4}$$

From equation 4 it can be appreciated that consumption is an estimate of global oxygen usage calculated using the difference in oxygen content in arterial and venous blood standardized to CO or the cardiac index (cardiac output in relation to body surface area).

At rest, given normal hemoglobin concentration and adequate cardiac output, oxygen delivery exceeds oxygen consumption levels with only 25% consumed of the total oxygen delivered. This number represents an average consumption of all tissues across the body. With adequate oxygen delivery, the central venous oxygen content ($ScvO_2$) is greater than 70%. When metabolic demand increases (e.g., fever, shivering), oxygen extraction increases, and central venous oxygen content may fall.

Oxygen extraction ratio (O_2ER) represents the amount or fraction of arterial oxygen content that is consumed as blood crosses across a tissue bed [2]. The equation for the oxygen extraction ratio is given below (Eq. 5) and is the difference between arterial O_2 content and venous O_2 content divided by arterial O_2 content

$$O_2ER = (CaO_2 - CvO_2)/CaO_2 \tag{5}$$

Normally, this ratio is around 0.2–0.3 which indicates the abundance of delivered oxygen [1]. The actual extraction ratio varies with different tissues depending on the basal metabolic rates. For instance, the brain and myocardial tissue extract the most oxygen when compared to other organs. Conversely, the kidney and liver extract the least oxygen. Tissues such as myocardial tissues are therefore more dependent on oxygen delivery and are more susceptible to ischemia as they are unable to extract more oxygen. Additionally, certain tissues can increase their oxygen extraction (e.g., skeletal muscles during heavy exercise) depending on changes in their metabolic demands.

Figure 2 summarizes the relationships between oxygen delivery consumption and extraction. As oxygen delivery falls, extraction rises in order to maintain a fixed consumption level required by tissues. With increased extraction, $ScvO_2$ begins to fall. Consumption is maintained by increasing oxygen extraction levels up until the critical point. This phase is termed the supply independent phase as a decrease in delivery will not

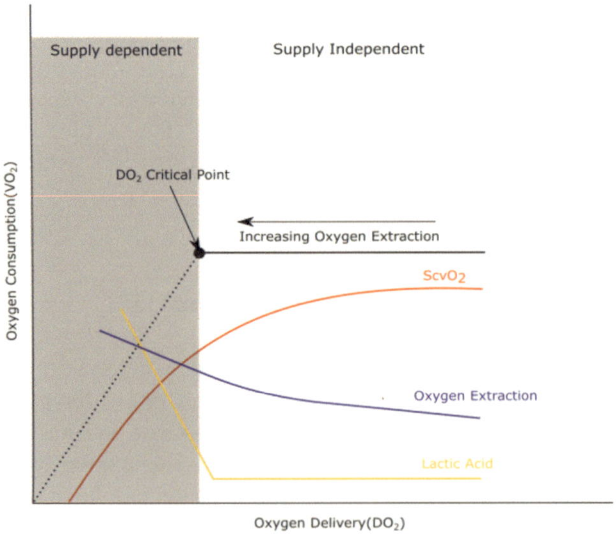

Figure 2.
Oxygen delivery and consumption relationship.

reduce consumption. Beyond the critical point, extraction can no longer maintain the cells metabolic demands and consumption begins to fall linearly with decreasing oxygen delivery. This phase is termed the supply dependent phase. In this phase ischemia sets in and lactic acid begins to accumulate due to oxygen deprivation and anaerobic respiration.

5. Pathophysiology and progression of shock

As previously defined, shock is a pathological state in which there is an imbalance in oxygen supply and demand. Ultimately it results in global hypoperfusion and a resulting increase in anaerobic respiration causing lactic acidosis (**Table 1**).

5.1 Compensated shock

When oxygen supply is inadequate, the body undergoes several physiological changes to maintain the oxygen delivery requirements and perfusion pressure. This stage is referred to as compensated shock and early signs of shock may be appreciated during this stage. Findings consistent with compensated shock are briefly mentioned in **Table 2**. At this point, it is important to identify the underlying cause and correct it to prevent any lasting complications. Homeostatic changes that occur are listen in **Table 1** and is stimulated by activation of two pathways. The first is **baroreceptor activation**. Decreased arterial pressure leads to decreased stretch of the baroreceptors located on the carotid sinus. There is a consequent decrease in afferent baroreceptor firing which increases efferent sympathetic firing and decreases efferent parasympathetic firing. Sympathetic activation results in an **increase in CO** via an increase in heart rate and stroke volume (increase in contractility). **Arteriolar vasoconstriction** allows for the redistribution of blood flow to more vital organs such as the brain, heart and kidneys. Additionally, increased sympathetic tone results in **constriction of venous circulation** thereby increasing venous return. As circulation is a closed system, an increase in venous return or preload brings about an increase in stroke volume and thereby cardiac output. Additionally, the sympathetic nervous system (SNS) directly stimulates the adrenal glands resulting in secretion of epinephrine, norepinephrine and cortisol which also aid in augmenting arteriolar and venous tone. The second pathway is activation of the **renin-angiotensin-aldosterone-system (RAAS).** A decrease in renal perfusion secondary to systemic hypotension triggers this activation. Aldosterone acts on the

Maintaining adequate circulating volume	*Vasoconstriction* via ↑ Sympathetic Tone, catecholamine release, angiotensin II release (RAAS) and vasopressin release
	Increased renal reabsorption via activation of RAAS and vasopressin release
Maximization of cardiac output	*Increase in heart rate*
	Increase in contractility
	↑*Preload* → ↑*CO* (Frank-Starling relationship)
Redirection of blood flow to vital organs	*Autoregulation* of blood flow to vital organs
Optimizing oxygen unloaded settings	↑*RBC 2-3-DPG* concentration
	Bohr Effect (lactic acidosis)

Table 1.
Compensatory mechanisms in response to systemic hypotension.

principal cells in the collecting tubules of the kidney to increase sodium reabsorption. This results in fluid retention that ultimately improves cardiac output. The angiotensin II acts on AT1 receptors on vascular endothelial cells causing vasoconstriction. Angiotensin II also preferentially constricts the efferent arteriole maintaining the glomerular filteration rate (GFR) and preventing pre-renal acute kidney injury in the setting of shock. These mechanisms briefly mentioned here all aim to maintain perfusion pressure, direct blood to vital organs (e.g. brain, heart, and kidney) and increase oxygen delivery in the setting of systemic hypoxia. A comprehensive table listing the various compensatory mechanisms in response to hypoxia is given (**Table 1**).

5.2 Uncompensated shock

When compensatory mechanisms are inadequate and DO_2 begins to fall beyond the critical point, shock has progressed to the **uncompensated stage**. During this stage there is rapid deterioration of the patient due to prolonged hypoxia and anaerobic respiration. When this state persists, a cascade of events occurs resulting in various pathophysiological outcomes outlined in **Figure 3**.

Lactic acid accumulation has an effect on several organs systems. Cardiac contractility has been shown to be reduced in states of acidosis further worsening DO_2. Acidosis also causes a predisposition to ventricular arrhythmias. At the cellular level, the function of pH dependent enzymes such as 6-phosphofructokinase, essential in glycolysis, are compromised further retarding ATP production. As hypoxia progresses, cells begin to deplete their ATP stores resulting in the dysfunction of various ATP dependent enzymatic reactions. Of key importance is the dysfunction of ion pumps which maintain membrane potential and cellular fluid dynamics. About 70 percent of ATP produced by cells is used to maintain sodium-potassium ATPase pumps. In the setting of hypoxemia there is decreased ATP production resulting in Na+/K+ ATPase pumps failure. Improper functioning ion pumps results in an influx of sodium and efflux of potassium altering the osmotic equilibrium between extracellular and intracellular fluids. This results in cellular edema leading to cell dysfunction and rupture. This is the underlying issue of all types of shock and leads to the most damaging outcome of hypoxia. Cellular hypoxia also activates monocytes which result in the release of cytokines. This triggers a cascade

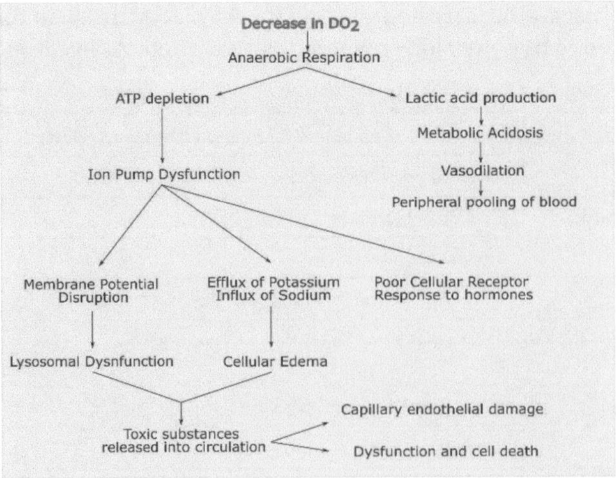

Figure 3.
Cellular response to hypoxia.

System	Compensated shock	Uncompensated shock
Neurological	Alert and oriented. Irritable	Altered mental status, Decreased responsiveness
Cardiovascular	Tachycardia	Tachycardia, Hypotension (MAP < 60 mmHg)
Respiratory	Tachypnea, Increased Work of Breathing*	Tachypnea, Decreased oxygen saturation, ARDS
Renal/GU	Decreased urine output (<0.5 mL/kg/h)	Prerenal azotemia, Metabolic acidosis, Anuria
Gastrointestinal	Nausea, Anorexia	Absence/Hypoactive bowel sounds, Ischemic bowel
Endocrine	Hyperglycemia	Hypoglycemia
Integumentary	Warm extremities with normal capillary refill time	Cold extremities with slow capillary refill time
Labs	Decreased venous PO_2	Elevated lactate

**Increased work of breathing is evident by findings such as subcostal recessions, sternal recession and nasal flaring.*

Table 2.
Findings in compensated and uncompensated shock.

ultimately leading to more vasodilation and increased vascular permeability further contributing to reduced tissue perfusion and hypotension. Additionally, lysosomal ion channel dysfunction disrupts lysosomal membrane potential leading to their dysfunction and release of contents. Both lysosome and cellular rupture lead to the release of toxic substances into extracellular fluids and circulation resulting in a cascade of capillary endothelial damage and cell death. Ultimately, these events produce findings such as hyperkalemia, hyponatremia, prerenal azotemia and lactic acidosis.

Clinical findings for both compensated and uncompensated shock are contrasted on **Table 2**.

5.3 Irreversible shock

The final stage of shock is irreversible shock which is also referred to as refractory shock. This final stage of shock carries a 96–99% mortality rate. There is loss of almost all compensatory mechanisms. Decreased perfusion exacerbates anaerobic metabolism processes due to lack of oxygen delivery to end-organs. Vasodilation and increased vascular permeability results in plasma leaving the vascular space, contributing to profound interstitial edema and loss of intravascular volume. This results in refractory hypotension, end organ ischemia, Multiple Organ Dysfunction Syndrome (MODS) and ultimately death.

6. Systemic inflammatory response syndrome (SIRS)

One complication that may arise as shock progresses is the development of **Systemic Inflammatory Response Syndrome (SIRS)**. While SIRS may not always be present in the progression of shock, its presence heralds the onset of a more serious syndrome mentioned earlier; Multiple Organ Dysfunction Syndrome (MODS). SIRS is defined as an "exaggerated defense response to a noxious stressor" and can be due to

Symptoms/Findings
Fever >100.4 F
Hypothermia <96.8 F
Tachypnea (Respiratory Rate > 20/min)
Tachycardia <90 bpm
WBC > 12,000/μL or WBC < 4000/μL
Bands >10%
Hyperglycemia >140 mg/dL with no DM*
*Diabetes Mellitus.

Table 3.
Diagnostic criteria for SIRS is the presence of any two of the above criteria.

insults such as infection, trauma, surgery, acute inflammation, and ischemia or reperfusion injury [3]. The relationship between shock and SIRS is not linear and one does not necessarily arise from the other. Shock may progress in the absence of SIRS depending on the etiology and type of shock. Infection is the most common cause of SIRS and is termed sepsis. In the early phases of septic shock, a cause of distributive shock discussed later, pathological stimuli result in cellular and immunological activation. This cellular activation leads to the release of a variety of chemokines including histamine, kinin, prostaglandins, leukotrienes and complement. Over activation of this system results in an imbalance between pro-inflammatory and anti-inflammatory mechanisms. Diagnostic criteria for determining SIRS are outlined in **Table 3**.

The outcomes of this imbalance occur globally, are a result of increased pro-inflammatory activity and are listed below:

a. Peripheral Vasodilation

b. Endothelial dysfunction ➔ Increase capillary permeability

c. Cellular activation ➔ neutrophils, macrophages, mast cells, platelets, endothelial cells

d. Microvascular coagulation ➔ end-organ micro thrombosis

e. Loss of circulatory integrity

7. Multiple organ dysfunction syndrome

Multiple Organ Dysfunction Syndrome (MODS) is a potentially life-threatening condition and is a major cause of high mortality in the intensive care unit reaching a range of 11–54% in septic pediatric patients [4]. It is defined as the 'development of potentially reversible physiological derangement involving two or more organ systems not involved in the disorder that resulted in ICU admission" and is a result of persisting states of shock, sepsis and hypoperfusion [4]. Most often, it is the end stage in the progression of septic shock and commonly affects the lungs, myocardium and brain before other organs. It is believed that the role of pro-inflammatory cytokines is key in inducing damage. Increased capillary leakage in the lungs causing pulmonary edema and surfactant loss, increased circulating nitrous oxide causing myocardial dysfunction and disturbances in the blood–brain barrier are all mechanisms thought to induce damage to these organs [4].

8. Types of shock

Shock can be broadly classified into four different types based on the pathological mechanism resulting in impaired oxygen delivery to the tissues. When dealing with a patient presenting with shock, it is important to identify the type of shock as all of them are treated differently. The four types of shock are:

1. Hypovolemic Shock

2. Cardiogenic Shock

3. Distributive Shock

4. Obstructive Shock

8.1 Hypovolemic shock

Hypovolemic shock occurs due to loss of intravascular volume. This is the most common type of shock. Loss of intravascular volume can be in the form of loss of blood or loss of fluids from the body other than blood. Causes of blood loss can include trauma, gastrointestinal bleeding, postpartum hemorrhage, esophageal varices and ruptured abdominal aortic aneurysm. Causes of non-blood fluid losses can include diarrhea, vomiting, reduced intake, third degree burns and diabetic ketoacidosis. Hypovolemic shock can be further classified according to the amount of volume loss. The classes of hypovolemic shock are given in **Table 4**.

8.2 Cardiogenic shock

Cardiogenic shock occurs due to inability of the heart to pump blood adequately to the peripheral circulation as a result of impaired contractility. This leads to end-organ

Class	Volume loss	Pulse	Blood pressure	Capillary refill	Respiratory rate	Urine output (mL/kg/h)
I	0–15%	Normal	Normal	Normal	Normal	1–2
II	15–30%	Mild Tachycardia	Mildly Low	Mildly Prolonged	Mild Tachypnea	0.5–1
III	30–40%	Tachycardia	Low	Prolonged	Tachypnea	0.25–0.5
IV	>40%	Tachycardia, Bradycardia or absent	Very Low	Greatly Prolonged	Severe Tachypnea	0

Table 4.
Classes of hypovolemic shock.

hypoxia and shock. Causes of cardiogenic shock can be myocardial infarction, myocarditis (secondary to Coxsackie B virus), dilated cardiomyopathy, and congenital heart disease, valvular dysfunction like aortic valve stenosis or mitral valve stenosis and arrhythmias. Both tachy-arrhythmias and brady-arrhythmias can lead to cardiogenic shock. Tachy-arrhythmias cause the heart to beat abnormally fast which impairs the filling ability of the heart, hence decreasing the preload and subsequently decreasing the cardiac output. Brady-arrhythmias decrease the heart rate and since CO = SV x HR, this also causes the cardiac output to decrease.

8.3 Distributive shock

Distributive shock occurs due to inappropriately distributed blood volume. Under normal physiology, vascular tone is under control of the autonomic nervous system. Sympathetic stimulation causes vascular smooth muscle to contract and vasoconstrict, while the parasympathetic nervous system causes vascular smooth muscle to relax and vasodilate. Distributive shock occurs when the sympathetic nervous system is unable to maintain the tone of the vascular system, allowing abnormal vasodilation of blood vessels. This allows pooling of blood and decreases preload. This also leads to increased vascular permeability and third-space fluid loss. This in turn causes intravascular hypovolemia and decreased end-organ perfusion. Distributive shock can have different etiologies like septic shock, anaphylactic shock and neurogenic shock.

Septic shock is the most common cause of distributive shock [5]. It can be defined as "sepsis-induced hypotension (systolic blood pressure <90 mm Hg or a reduction of 40 mm Hg from baseline) despite adequate fluid resuscitation along with the presence of perfusion abnormalities that may include, but are not limited to, lactic acidosis, oliguria, or an acute alteration in mental status." Septic shock results from an overwhelming systemic inflammatory response which leads to vasodilation and subsequent hypotension. Most common causes of septic shock are gram negative bacteria like *Escherichia coli*, Proteus species, *Klebsiella pneumoniae* which release endotoxins which are responsible for activation of the immune system.

Anaphylactic shock occurs due to type 1 hypersensitivity reaction to any foreign antigen. Antigens bind to IgE molecules on pre-sensitized mast cells and cause mast cell degranulation and release of inflammatory mediators like histamine. Histamine causes vasodilation and increased capillary permeability. This causes severe hypovolemia and cardiovascular collapse leading to shock.

Neurogenic shock results from the inability of the sympathetic nervous system to maintain the tone of blood vessels. In most cases, this is a result of trauma to the brain or spinal cord above the level of T6 [6]. The trauma leads to a loss of background sympathetic stimulation to the vascular smooth muscles. This causes vasodilation resulting in a sudden decrease in blood pressure (secondary to a decrease in peripheral vascular resistance).

8.4 Obstructive shock

Obstructive shock occurs when there is a barrier to the flow of blood or a barrier which impairs proper filling of the heart. There are several conditions which can cause obstructive shock. These include cardiac tamponade, tension pneumothorax and pulmonary embolism.

Cardiac tamponade is the result of fluid in the pericardial space which impairs the filling ability of the heart during diastole. This reduces the preload and subsequently decreases cardiac output. This is similar in presentation to constrictive pericarditis in which the pericardium shrinks and hardens.

Tension pneumothorax is the presence of air in the pleural cavity under positive pressure. The elevated intrathoracic pressure leads to decreased venous return to the heart as it compresses the inferior vena cava, thus leading to reduced cardiac output.

Pulmonary embolism is an embolus (usually dislodged from the proximal deep veins of the lower limb) lodged in the vasculature of the lungs. This obstructs blood flowing to the lungs and the blood coming from the lungs to the heart. There is a decrease in end-diastolic volume which leads to a decreased stroke volume and hence decreased cardiac output and oxygen delivery to the peripheral tissues resulting in shock.

9. Resuscitation goals

When approaching a patient in shock, management requires attaining physiological normalcy and hemodynamic stability. In the clinical setting, the progress of treatment is measured by achieving certain goals. These clinical goals help ascertain improvement in global perfusion and oxygenation. Factors measured are included in **Table 5** and are used clinically to determine a patient's response to the management of shock. While these conditions are useful in measuring response, the use of only one or two as an indicator for improvement will lead to shortcomings and mislead a physician regarding the actual response to management.

One goal used to assess treatment is normalcy in heart rate and perfusion pressure representing adequate perfusion and venous return/cardiac output. Perfusion pressure is determined by subtracting the central venous pressure (CVP) by the mean arterial pressure (MAP); MAP-CVP. These parameters can be used to measure hemodynamic stability and are also used to assess response to fluid therapy. With administration of a fluid bolus, heart rate should ideally decrease and MAP-CVP should increase. Another measurement that can be used to assess response to fluid therapy and inotrope therapy response is the shock index (HR/SBP). Calculated by dividing

Indicators of therapeutic responsiveness	Normal value/Prognostic value
Normal Mental Status	GCS = 15/15
Normal pulse quality and rate	Palpable in all extremities; Rate varies with age
Difference in Central and peripheral temperatures	36.1–37.2°C; equal centrally and peripherally
Normal Capillary Refill	≤ 2 seconds
Adequate Urine Output	>1 mL/kg/h
Lactate Trends	≥0.75 mmol/L/h. associated with bad prognosis
Normal Superior Vena Cava Oxygen Saturation (SVC O_2)	≥ 70%
$AVDO_2$	≤5 mL O_2/100 mL of blood

Table 5.
Resuscitative goals and normal values.

heart rate (HR) by systolic blood pressure (SPB), the shock index should ideally decrease as fluid therapy is directed at improving stroke volume, thereby decreasing HR, and inotrope therapy improves vascular tone and SBP.

As mentioned earlier, during shock states compensatory mechanisms redirect blood to vital organs such as the brain, heart and kidneys. Consequently, as shock progresses from compensated to uncompensated phase, these organs will begin to show signs of dysfunction. Mental status of a patient is therefore a parameter which should be assessed to determine improvement in a patient's condition. While improvement is a good sign, not all patients will have altered mental status and, when present, is often a late manifestation of shock. Relying on altered mental status as an indicator of shock and its improvement as good response to therapy is not a reliable approach and should be taken with caution and in combination with other factors. The kidney is another organ which can be used to assess response to therapy. A normal urine output of >1 mL/kg/h represents adequate renal perfusion and perfusion pressure. However, urine output only represents the improvement in renal perfusion and does not provide a picture of global perfusion status.

Systemic vascular tone and cardiac output can both be determined by assessing peripheral temperatures, capillary refill and distal pulse qualities. Normal capillary refill is <2 seconds and coupled with normal peripheral temperature and distal pulses correlates with adequate perfusion to the peripheries. However, these parameters do not provide indication of oxygenation. Cases such as anemia or hemodilution may have normal peripheral temperature, pulses and capillary refill but oxygen delivery is still impaired.

As shock is defined as impaired systemic oxygen delivery, lactate levels are a good indicator of global oxygenation. Lactate trends should be observed rather than single serum lactate measurements as a single measurement does not indicate the progression of disease. Increases of lactate levels of ≥ 70 mmol/L/h. is associated with worsening oxygen delivery and outcomes.

Superior vena cava oxygen saturation ($SVCO_2$) of $\geq 70\%$ is a good therapeutic endpoint in the management of shock. As mentioned earlier in the chapter, when there is good oxygen delivery, $SVCO_2$ should be maintained above 70% representing no increase in oxygen extraction during the compensatory phase of shock. Measuring $SVCO_2$ can be done via central venous catheters with venous oximetry or, more recently, with the use of near-infrared spectroscopy, a less invasive method. One can also calculate the difference in arterial and venous oxygen content ($AVDO_2$) to assess the degree of oxygen extraction during this phase of shock. Normal values show a difference of ≤ 5 mL O_2/100 mL of blood and increases in $AVDO_2$ indicate increases in oxygen extraction.

10. General principles in the treatment of shock

In order to provide a patient with the benefit of rational and effective treatment, it is critical to identify the specific cause of shock in each case. Although treatment should be aimed at the underlying etiology of shock, the most critical aspect of treatment is the prompt restoration of normal hemodynamics.

From a hemodynamic perspective, there are three main categories in the management of shock:

- Intravenous fluids, which act by increasing central venous pressure and downstream left ventricular end-diastolic volume (EDV)
- Vasopressors which act by increase systemic vascular resistance (SVR)
- Inotropes which act by increasing contractility and thus increase cardiac output

In hypovolemic shock, the primary derangement is low central venous pressure (CVP) so therefore IV fluids are the cornerstone of therapy. If the patient is profoundly hypotensive, vasopressors are sometimes used temporarily but only while definitive access is obtained, and fluids are pushed as quickly as possible. If a patient in hypovolemic shock is requiring vasopressors to maintain enough perfusion pressure to stay conscious, they are in critical need for more fluid. Since these patients are already extremely hyper dynamic, there are no benefits of inotropes which will only risk worsening tachycardia to the point that diastolic filling time is too short for the left ventricle to fill.

In distributive shock, the primary derangement is low SVR. Vasopressors are therefore almost always necessary. Since most of these patients are also hypovolemic, or at the very least, have fluid maldistributed to the extravascular space rather than central circulation, IV fluids are also used in every case. Because of sepsis induced cardiomyopathy, some patients with sepsis may also benefit from inotropes but identifying those patients can be a challenge.

In cardiogenic shock, the primary problem is low cardiac output, thus inotropes are the mainstay therapy. Both fluids and vasopressors are not only unnecessary but contraindicated. In fact, reduction in preload by using diuretics, and reducing the afterload helps in augmenting the cardiac output in patients with cardiogenic shock.

Finally, in obstructive shock, it is impossible to generalize about the appropriateness of fluids, vasopressors and inotropes and if there is a response to any of those, it is likely only temporary. Definitive relief of the obstruction is still critical. For pneumothorax (PTX), this is either chest tube or needle thoracostomy which consists of a needle placed into the pleural space via the second intercostal space in the midclavicular line. For cardiac tamponade, pericardiocentesis can be performed, a procedure in which a needle is placed in the pericardial space most commonly via a subxiphoid approach. In case of massive pulmonary embolism, depending on the circumstances, this may require systemic thrombolysis or embolectomy.

General treatment principles are summarized in **Table 6**.

Type of shock	IV Fluids (↑CVP)	Vasopressors (↑SVR)	Inotropes (↑Contractility)
Hypovolemic	+	Temporary use only	–
Distributive	+	+	+/–
Cardiogenic	–	–	+
Obstructive	+/–	+/–	+/–

Table 6.
General approach to therapy with regards to type of shock.

10.1 Fluid therapy

Fluid resuscitation is the rapid delivery of fluids to patients who have acutely impaired hemodynamics. Resuscitative fluids are given universally to patients in hypovolemic shock and lesser forms of dehydration, as well as to almost all patients with severe sepsis and septic shock. In these situations, the preload to the heart is not enough for adequate cardiac output. To understand why these patients are given fluids we need to review the Frank-Starling curve as shown in **Figure 4**. According to the Frank-Starling Law, the length of myocardial tissue is directly related to the force of the subsequent contraction. The more myocardial fibers are stretched, the more they contract. Preload determines the degree of myocardial fiber stretching. Therefore, as shown in **Figure 4**, an increase in preload results in a responsive increase in stroke volume. Patients on the left side of the curve are those who are preload dependent. Towards the right, the curve flattens and increases in preload are met with a reduced rate of increase in stroke volume until we see no change in stoke volume with increasing preload. These patients are preload independent. Essentially, only if the patient is preload dependent will we see benefits to stroke volume if given fluid. Preload independent patients will not benefit from fluids. It is important to note that the shape and position of the curve will vary between individuals, and it is important to identify where on the curve the patient lies to determine whether it is suitable to give fluids.

Once we have decided which patient needs to be given fluids, we need to decide which fluids to give. The first decision to make is whether to give crystalloid or colloid. Crystalloids are fluids which contain water and various electrolytes and other small water-soluble molecules. Colloids are large, insoluble molecules and oftentimes proteins. Theoretically, colloid should be superior to crystalloid as it has an increased tendency to stay intravascular. However, a 2013 Cochrane review found no evidence from randomized controlled trials that resuscitation with colloids reduces the risk of death, compared to resuscitation with crystalloids, in patients with trauma, burns or following surgery [7]. Therefore, given their decreased cost and increased availability,

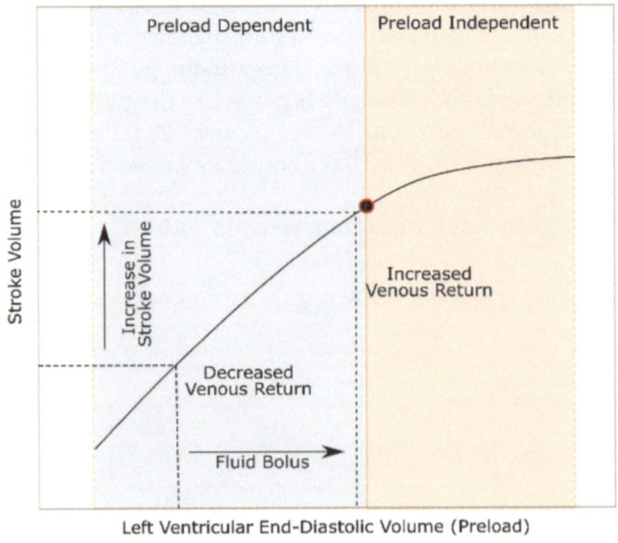

Figure 4.
Frank-Starling curve.

as well as the low immunogenic response, crystalloids are almost always favored over colloids.

Crystalloid replacement is usually sufficient in hypovolemic shock caused by vomiting and diarrhea. The presence or absence of associated electrolyte disturbances (e.g., hypo- or hypernatremia) determines the type of crystalloid. The use of albumin as a replacement fluid for hypovolemic shock is probably best reserved for situations involving direct albumin loss (e.g., burns, open wounds, protein-losing enteropathies). Volume replacement with crystalloid or albumin may be appropriate in cases of hemorrhagic shock, but with significant blood loss, replacement of red blood cell mass will eventually become necessary.

While the majority of patients with hypovolemic shock tolerate relatively rapid correction of intravascular volume depletion, there are a few notable exceptions that may require slower correction. For example, in cases of hypovolemic shock accompanied by significant metabolic/electrolyte derangements (e.g., hypernatremia or diabetic ketoacidosis), volume deficit correction must be tempered so that the accompanying metabolic/electrolyte abnormalities are not corrected too quickly. Rapid correction of hypernatremia can lead to cerebral edema while rapid correction of hyponatremia can lead to central pontine myelinolysis.

Correction of hypovolemic shock in patients with underlying myocardial dysfunction must be done with greater caution than in patients with normal myocardial function to avoid further compromising myocardial function. Finally, in trauma-specific situations, very aggressive volume resuscitation for hemorrhagic shock may not be appropriate until surgical hemorrhage control is achieved.

10.2 Blood products

Oxygen delivery, as described in the first section, is dependent on two factors: cardiac output and arterial oxygen content. Vasoactive and fluid therapy both aim to enhance cardiac output and global perfusion to enhance oxygen deliver. In both these therapies the arterial oxygen content remains the same. The use of blood products aims to increase arterial oxygen content (CaO_2) by infusing packed red blood cells (PRBC) thereby increasing hemoglobin levels, the main parameter determining arterial oxygen content. The use of PRBC is therefore most useful in situations where shock is caused or worsened by decreasing hemoglobin concentration such as in patients with hemolytic anemia. The goal of blood product therapy is to return hemoglobin concentrations to normal values with regards to age. Approximately 10 mL/kg of PRBC should increase hemoglobin concentration by 2 g/dL. A 20 kg child with an Hb concentration of 5 g/dL would therefore require 500 mL of PRBC to reach an Hb concentration of 10 g/dL. When considering blood transfusion, it is important to consider the hemodynamic changes that occur with increasing hematocrit. Experimentally it has been shown that a hematocrit of 30% is optimal for oxygen delivery while hematocrit levels exceeding 40% increase viscosity and hinder oxygen delivery [8].

10.3 Vasoactive therapy

Vasoactive drugs used in the management of shock can be divided into inotropic, vasoconstrictive and vasodilative medication. The main goals of employing these medications are to increase cardiac output, decrease vascular resistance and increase perfusion pressure. The administration of these drugs usually come after initial use of fluid and blood product therapies fail to produce adequate improvement.

Inotropes: Inotropes are generally used to increase cardiac output and stroke volume. Their mechanism of action usually involves stimulation of adrenergic receptors and includes endogenous catecholamines such as dopamine, epinephrine and norepinephrine and exogenous catecholamines such as dobutamine and phenylephrine. These drugs work to stimulate α-adrenergic, β-adrenergic and dopaminergic receptors which subsequently alter conditions such as contractility and systemic vascular resistance (vasodilation or vasoconstriction) thereby influencing cardiac output and perfusion pressures. In the setting of shock, the use of these drugs helps enhance cardiac function to improve oxygen delivery.

Aside from drugs such as phenylephrine, most inotropic drugs will stimulate multiple receptor types with varying selectivity. For example, as shown in **Table 7**, dopamine will preferentially stimulate dopaminergic receptors but will also stimulate β- and α-adrenergic receptors and will therefore exhibit varying and multiple physiological changes in a dose dependent manner. It is therefore important to know drugs selectivity and the physiological response of each receptor type. **β_1-adrenergic receptors** are primary expressed in myocardial tissue and have positive inotropic and chronotropic activity when stimulated. Stimulation of this receptor directly enhances cardiac output by increasing heart rate and contractility (stroke volume). **β_2-adrenergic receptors** act on smooth muscle of vascular tissue and bronchial tissue and produce vasodilation and bronchodilation respectively. **α_1-adrenergic receptors** work mainly on vascular smooth muscles contraction and cause peripheral vasoconstriction. **α_2-adrenergic receptors** one the other hand causes vasodilation via the inhibition of norepinephrine secretion from presynaptic sympathetic neurons. **Dopaminergic receptors (DA)** receptors act on renal vasculature and causing renal arterial vasodilation.

Dopamine, in terms of inotropic therapy, displays dose-dependent activity on dopaminergic, β- and α-adrenergic receptors. At low doses (0-3 μg/kg/min) dopamine acts as a mild vasodilator in peripheral vasculature by stimulating the release of norepinephrine [9]. Additionally, it inhibits norepinephrine reuptake in presynaptic sympathetic neurons indirectly enhancing contractility and heart rate [9]. Activation of dopaminergic receptors at low doses also improves renal and splanchnic perfusion via D_2 presynaptic receptors potentially providing renal protective activity [8, 9], but it remains matter of debate. Stimulation of D_2 presynaptic receptors enhances vasodilation in coronary, renal, mesenteric and cerebral vasculature promoting improved blood flow to these organs [9]. While inhibition of norepinephrine reuptake in sympathetic neurons does have vasoconstrictive activity, the direct vasodilatory effects in peripheral vasculature offsets the level of constriction resulting in mild elevation of SVR. Ultimately, dopamine has the combined effect of significantly improving contractility and heart rate with only mild changes in SVR resulting in effective improvement in cardiac output. At higher doses (>10 μg/kg/min) α-adrenergic activity is stimulated causing vasoconstriction and aids in increasing blood pressure [8, 9].

Epinephrine is a nonselective catecholamine stimulating both adrenergic receptors of all types. Therefore, is produces both increases in CO and increases in SVR. When administered at a low dose at an infusion rate of 0.03–0.3 μg/kg/min, epinephrine mostly exhibits inotropic activity via β-adrenergic receptors increasing cardiac output. As higher infusion rates >0.3 μg/kg/min are used, α-adrenergic activity is also activated resulting in vasoconstriction and an increase in SVR. Because of its selective inotropic activity at low doses, epinephrine is reliable choice in patients with hypotension without myocardial dysfunction. In high doses epinephrine has also been seen to cause atrial and ventricular arrhythmias [9]. One aspect of inotropic therapy using epinephrine is its administration in correlation with elevated lactate levels. Studies have shown that epinephrine may elevate lactate levels, interfering with lactate trends. It is therefore important to interpret lactate trends with skepticism when assessing response to therapy and concomitant resuscitation goals should be viewed when using epinephrine.

Norepinephrine preferentially binds α_1-adrenergic receptors over β-adrenergic receptors resulting in more vasoconstrictive activity than inotropic activity. Because of its potent α-receptor stimulation, norepinephrine is the vasopressor drug of choice in distributive shock with hypotension [9]. At low doses of 0.01–0.05 μg/kg/min its inotropic activity can be appreciated with an improvement in cardiac output. However, at higher doses, its affinity for α-adrenergic receptors takes over, vastly increasing vasoconstriction and blood pressure. This shift in receptor activity can impede cardiac output especially in patients with cardiac dysfunction.

Dobutamine is a synthetic catecholamine that has mixed β- and α-adrenergic stimulation at varying dosages. It primary acts as an inotrope increasing contractility with minimal increases in SVR indicating its use in patients with cardiogenic shock. Additionally, at infusion rates >10 μg/kg/min dobutamine can reduce afterload by stimulating α_2-adrenergic stimulation causing vasodilation [8]. In this setting dobutamine can improve cardiac output [8]. At low doses of <5 μg/kg/min, dobutamine can exhibit α_1-aderenergic antagonism resulting in vasodilation and decreased afterload.

Phenylephrine is a pure α_1-adrengeric agonist and has strong vasoconstrictor activity. It can be used as an additional therapy where an increase in vascular tone is needed without changes in cardiac function.

Phosphodiesterase inhibitors (Milrinone) work as an inotrope via a different mechanism than the catecholamines described above. By inhibiting phosphodiesterase, it causes an increase in intracellular cAMP levels thereby increasing intracellular Ca^{2+}. These changes subsequently increase both inotropic activity in myocytes and

Drug	Receptor/mechanism	Effect
Dopamine	Dopaminergic (DA) > β-adrenergic > α-adrenergic	Low doses (DA) → ↑renal artery vasodilation
		Mod/high. Doses (DA + β) → ↑renal blood flow, HR, contractility, CO
Dobutamine	α- & β-adrenergic	↑CO with minimal effects on BP
Epinephrine	α_1 & β-adrenergic	↑SVR, HR, CO, BP
Phenylephrine	Pure α_1-adrenergic	Peripheral arterial vasoconstriction → ↑BP, MAP, SVR
Norepinephrine	Mixed α_1 & β-adrenergic ($\alpha_1 > \beta_1 > \beta_2$)	Significant ↑BP + MAP, SVR, CO, HR
Vasopressin	V-1 & V-2 receptors	↑BP, SVR; anti-diuretic action via V-2
Phosphodiesterase Inhibitor (Milrinone)	↑cAMP	↑CO + vasodilation → ↓BP

Table 7.
Mechanism of action and effects of inotropes and vasopressors.

vasodilation in vascular smooth muscle. It has the advantage of achieving these results without acting on adrenergic receptors and is therefore ideal in situations where receptor downregulation has developed due to chronic inotrope usage such as in those patients with chronic heart failure [9].

Vasopressin maintains perfusion pressure through two main mechanisms. Firstly, it acts on blood vessels to produce vasoconstriction via the activation of V_1-receptors. This causes an increase in SVR and thereby increases arterial pressure. Secondly, it stimulates V_2-receptors on renal tubular cells to enhance fluid reabsorption via aquaporin channels. Vasopressin is also known to stimulate CRH release from the hypothalamus, thereby increasing downstream ACTH and cortisol secretion. Cortisol in turn enhances vasoconstriction and inhibits secretion of vasodilators such as PGE2 and nitric oxide.

Mechanisms of these drugs and their effect on the cardiovascular system are summarized in **Table 7**.

Author details

Numair Belgaumi, Ahmed Salik and Naveed ur Rehman Siddiqui*
The Aga Khan University Hospital, Medical College, Pakistan

*Address all correspondence to: naveed.rehman@aku.edu

References

[1] Lucking SE, Maffei FA, Tamburro RF, Zaritsky A, editors. Pediatric Critical Care: Text and Study Guide. 2nd ed. Cham, Switzerland: Springer Nature; 2021. pp. 27-48

[2] Taha M, Elbaih A. Pathophysiology and management of different types of shock. Narayana Medical Journal. 2017;**6**: 14-39

[3] Chakraborty RKBB. Systemic Inflammatory Response Syndrome [Internet]. Treasure Island, Florida: In: StatPearls. Treasure Island (FL): StatPearls Publishing; 2020;2020. Available from: https://www.ncbi.nlm.nih.gov/books/NBK547669/

[4] Ramírez M. Multiple organ dysfunction syndrome. Current Problems in Pediatric and Adolescent Health Care. 2013;**43**(10):273-277

[5] Martí-Carvajal AJ, Solà I, Gluud C, Lathyris D, Anand V. Human recombinant protein C for severe sepsis and septic shock in adult and paediatric patients. Cochrane Libr [Internet]. 2012: 5. DOI: 10.1002/14651858.cd004388.pub6

[6] Dilaveri CA. Perioperative medicine: Managing for outcome. In: Mayo Clinic Proceedings. 2009

[7] Perel P, Roberts I. Colloids versus crystalloids for fluid resuscitation in critically ill patients. Hoboken, New Jersey: John Wiley and Sons, Cochrane Database Syst Rev [Internet]. 2012;(6): CD000567. DOI: 10.1002/14651858.CD000567.pub5

[8] VanValkinburgh D, Kerndt CC, Hashmi MF. Inotropes and Vasopressors. StatPearls Publishing; 2021

[9] Kislitsina ON, Rich JD, Wilcox JE, Pham DT, Churyla A, Vorovich EB, et al. Shock–classification and pathophysiological principles of therapeutics. Current Cardiology Reviews. 2019;**15**(2):102-113

Chapter 3

Spinal Shock: Clinical Pearls

Sri Rama Ananta Nagabhushanam Padala, Vaishali Waindeskar, Ved Prakash Maurya, Rakesh Mishra and Amit Agrawal

Abstract

Spinal shock is a clinical manifestation following injury to the spinal cord resulting from multiple mechanisms. It is a complex phenomenon with flaccid paralysis, absent anal wink, and bulbocavernosus reflex. Management strategy for such patients includes rapid evaluation and treatment strategies to minimize the impact of secondary spinal cord injury. The advanced trauma life support (ATLS) guidelines provide the basis for rapid assessment and stabilization of A (Airway), B (Breathing), and C (Circulation) before dealing with the neurological deficits under the primary survey. The emergence of better radiological investigations has been pivotal in categorizing spinal syndromes and reaching a precise diagnosis. Early initiation of treatment measures results in better neurological and functional recovery with minimal residual deficits. The role of steroids in spinal shock has been a highly debated topic, and the timing of surgery is variable, intending to eliminate the secondary injury. Clinical differentiation between neurogenic and hypovolemic shock is vital, enhancing the quality of care with realistic outcome expectations.

Keywords: spinal shock, sympathetic, spinal injury, spinal reflex, spinal cord

1. Introduction

The term "spinal shock" was introduced to differentiate arterial hypotension, which is due to hemorrhage. Spinal shock appears following spinal cord injury leading to loss of sympathetic tone which is described in literature for more than 150 years [1–3]. This shock manifests as transient loss or impairment of all or part of spinal reflex activity below the level of the spinal injury that may be due to physiologic or anatomic transection of the spinal cord [4]. In this chapter, we review the basic concepts in the development of spinal shock, clinical presentations, management strategies, follow-up, and outcomes in patients with spinal shock.

1.1 Overview

In a majority of the cases, spinal shock result secondary to trauma (motor vehicle accidents, falls, sporting accidents, and self-harm) [5] causing either transection, hemorrhage, or ischemic injury to the spinal cord [6], other less-common causes include mechanical cord compression, hypotension, and hypoxia [7]. In spinal shock, descending facilitation of upper motor neurons in spinal cord injury patients is impaired, leading to difficulties differentiating upper motor neuron lesions from lower motor neuron lesions [8]. The somatic component of spinal shock and autonomic reflexes are variably affected depending on the level of injury and phase of recovery [8]. Clinically, the spinal shock is characterized by reversible and temporary loss of all neurological function (that includes motor and sensory dysfunction, variably depressed reflexes, detrusor and rectal tone) below a particular spinal level [6, 9–12]. During the recovery phase, acute loss of functions is followed by the development of spasticity with increased muscle tone, exaggerated deep tendon reflexes, and muscle spasms [13]. Usually, reflex detrusor contractility returns if the distal portions of the spinal cord are not damaged but rather isolated from higher centers. Initially, such reflex activity is not maintained correctly and the return of reflex bladder activity typically occurs with the recovery of deep tendon reflexes in the lower extremities [8].

2. Clinical evaluation

Resuscitation, hemodynamic stabilization, and clinical assessment of a patient with spinal shock are a simultaneous and ongoing process [4, 8]. Clinical details include a detailed history of the mode and mechanism of injury (hit by another vehicle, fall, rollover crash, ejection outside the car, or seat belt was used or not), any history of alcohol intoxication, history of any comorbid conditions, and a detailed spine and physical examination of all the systems to exclude any associated injuries or dysfunctions [14]. Neurological examination includes assessment of the level of consciousness, motor and sensory functions, and assessment of deep tendon and superficial reflexes [15–17]. This will help determine the lesion's level and the extent of neurological impairment. Additionally, attention should be paid to determine the associated autonomic dysfunction (including bowel and bladder disturbance), autonomic dysreflexia, and the presence and extent of cardiovascular dysfunctions [18]. Involvement of the respiratory system, particularly intercostal muscles and diaphragm, can result in respiratory compromise. Early recognition and appropriate intervention (elective ventilation, early tracheostomy), including chest physiology, will help recover respiratory functions.

2.1 Spinal shock versus neurogenic shock

Although "spinal shock" and "neurogenic shock" are used interchangeably to optimize the outcome, there is a need to identify these two entities separately. Neurogenic shock is characterized by the hemodynamic changes resulting from spinal cord injury (above T6) and a loss of autonomic tone resulting in hypotension and bradycardia [4]. In a broader perspective, neurogenic shock is a distributive shock characterized by hypotension, bradycardia, and peripheral vasodilatation. It can manifest following a significant central nervous system damage (head injury, cervical spinal cord, or high thoracic cord injuries) [4]. **Table 1** shows a comparative description of these two types of shock, frequently encountered in trauma patients [19–22]. In clinical practice, early identification of spinal shock relieves the patient's anxiety and better prognostication of the sequela following spine injury.

	Spinal shock	Neurogenic shock
Location of injury	Due to spinal cord injury at any level	Due to head injury and spinal cord injury at cervical and high thoracic spine (above T6) level
Onset	Sudden to days	Sudden
Mechanism	Temporary unresponsiveness of peripheral neurons to brain stimuli leads to loss of reflex activity below the level of lesion	Autonomic pathways disruption leads to loss of sympathetic tone and vasodilation
Affects	Just spinal cord is affected	Entire nervous system is affected
Clinical presentation	Clinically present as flaccidity followed by spasticity at a later stage	Clinically present as instability of blood pressure, heart rate, and temperature regulation
Systemic hypotension	Possible	Always
Treatment	No specific treatment for spinal shock	Phenylephrine/norepinephrine to regain the sympathetic tone and atropine/glycopyrrolate for bradycardia
Resolution	Usually a temporary phenomenon, recovering within 24 to 48 hours, but can persist for 4 weeks to months	Usually short

Table 1.
Comparison between spinal shock and neurogenic shock.

2.2 Management

In the majority, spinal shock is associated with traumatic spinal cord injuries and requires a comprehensive interprofessional team approach (consisting of emergency teams, neurosurgeons, neuro-rehabilitation experts, and social workers). Imaging evaluation includes magnetic resonance imaging (MRI) and a detailed spinal computed tomogram (CT) with bony details. Before performing the detailed imaging, initial evaluation, and management follow the protocol to manage any patient who presents to the emergency room and manage "Airway, Breathing and Circulation" [23]. These patients may need intubation, mechanical ventilation, central venous access, invasive monitoring, and vasopressors to manage hemodynamic instability and neurogenic shock. They may require management of the source of hemorrhage, pneumothorax, myocardial injury, pericardial tamponade, or any other source of hypotension [23, 24]. Patients with a high cervical injury who present with spinal shock shall need special attention as these may frequently require cardiovascular interventions, including pacemakers for symptomatic bradycardia [25]. Elective ventilation or early tracheostomy to prevent or manage respiratory complications [26]. These patients shall need nutritional support, prophylaxis to prevent gastric ulcers, deep vein thrombosis, a long-term indwelling urinary catheter for bladder dysfunction, toilet training for bowel dysfunction, and care from preventing pressure ulcers [6, 7].

2.3 Outcome

Although there is improved survival in the patients, the severity of neurological deficits determines the overall outcome of these patients [6–8]. Overall, spinal cord injury and shock are associated with poorer functional and overall outcomes requiring long-term rehabilitation care [15, 27].

2.4 Respiratory

The level of spinal cord injury usually determines the degree of respiratory support required in these patients. Complete injury above the level of C3 results in apneic respiratory arrest and death in the absence of prompt ventilatory support. Less-severe ventilatory impairment is associated with injuries below the C5 vertebra with various levels of respiratory failure for injuries between C3 and C5.

2.5 Cardiovascular

Involvement of cardiac accelerator fibers (T1–T4) is the cause of bradycardia and decreased myocardial contractility in these patients, often resulting in systemic hypotension and subsequent reduced spinal cord perfusion.

2.6 Deep venous thrombosis

Venous thromboembolism is one of the major causes of death, in addition to infectious complications after spinal cord injury. Antithrombotic prophylaxis by means of low molecular weight heparin or low-dose unfractionated heparin along with non-pharmacologic devices is helpful.

2.7 Gastrointestinal

There is increased risk of stress ulcers and upper gastrointestinal bleeds in these patients especially in those who are on mechanical ventilation and receiving high-dose steroids.

2.8 Neuropsychiatric

Depression, anxiety disorders, substance-related disorders, and suicidal tendencies are neuropsychiatric complications in these patients. Psychological support and counseling are essential.

Ditunno et al. [6]. described the loss of reflexes and recovery patterns in spinal shock patients in much detail depending upon duration following injury. He recognized four phases (Phase I–IV), phase I (Areflexia/hyporeflexia) postinjury day 0–1, phase II (Initial reflexes return) postinjury days 1–3, and phase III (Initial hyper-reflexia) postinjury between days 4 and 1 month and phase IV (Final hyperreflexia) occurs between 1 and 12-months after injury.

3. Conclusions

In patients with spinal injuries, spinal shock is associated with poor outcomes. In a case of a history of trauma, careful attention should be paid to recognizing the spinal injuries and reasonable efforts need to be made to avoid the aggravation of injuries. Management needs to focus on airway and respiratory dysfunction, hypotension, and cardiovascular abnormalities. Imaging modalities, including CT and MRI, can help identify the extent and type of injuries and expedite the decision to facilitate spinal cord decompression and stabilization as required.

Conflict of interest

The authors have no conflict of interest to declare.

Author details

Sri Rama Ananta Nagabhushanam Padala[1], Vaishali Waindeskar[1], Ved Prakash Maurya[2], Rakesh Mishra[3] and Amit Agrawal[4]*

1 Department of Anesthesia and Critical Care, All India Institute of Medical Sciences, Bhopal, India

2 Department of Neurosurgery, Sanjay Gandhi Post Graduate Institute of Medical Sciences, Lucknow, India

3 Department of Neurosurgery, Institute of Medical Sciences, Trauma Centre and Mahamana Centenary Superspeciality Hospital Banaras Hindu University, Varanasi, India

4 Department of Neurosurgery, All India Institute of Medical Sciences, Bhopal, India

*Address all correspondence to: dramitagrawal@gmail.com; dramitagrawal@hotmail.com

References

[1] Bastian HC. On the symptomatology of total transverse lesions of the spinal cord; with special reference to the condition of the various reflexes. Medico-Chirurgical Transactions. 1890;**73**:151-217. DOI: 10.1177/095952879007300113

[2] Hall M. On the diseases and derangements of the nervous system. In: Their Primary Forms and in their Modifications by Age, Sex, Constitution, Hereditary Predisposition, Excesses, General Disorder, and Organic Disease. Books on Demand. London: H. Bailliere; 1841

[3] Hall M. Synopsis of the Diastaltic Nervous System. London: Mallett; 1850

[4] Atkinson PP, Atkinson JL. Spinal shock. Mayo Clinic Proceedings. Apr 1996;**71**(4):384-389. DOI: 10.4065/71.4.384. PMID: 8637263

[5] Hall M. Second memoir on some principles of the pathology of the nervous system. Medico-Chirurgical Transactions. 1840;**23**:121

[6] Ditunno JF, Little JW, Tessler A, Burns AS. Spinal shock revisited: A four-phase model. Spinal Cord. 2004;**42**(7):383-395. DOI: 10.1038/sj.sc.3101603

[7] Sekhon LH, Fehlings MG. Epidemiology, demographics, and pathophysiology of acute spinal cord injury. Spine (Phila Pa 1976). 2001;**26** (24 Suppl):S2-S12. DOI: 10.1097/00007632-200112151-00002

[8] Ko HY. Revisit spinal shock: Pattern of reflex evolution during spinal shock. Korean Journal of Neurotrauma. 2018;**14**(2):47-54. DOI: 10.13004/kjnt.2018.14.2.47

[9] Biering-Sorensen F, Biering-Sorensen T, Liu N, Malmqvist L, Wecht JM, Krassioukov A. Alterations in cardiac autonomic control in spinal cord injury. Autonomic Neuroscience. 2018;**209**:4-18. DOI: 10.1016/j.autneu.2017.02.004

[10] Ketchum JM, Cuthbert JP, Deutsch A, et al. Representativeness of the spinal cord injury model systems National Database. Spinal Cord. 2018;**56**(2):126-132. DOI: 10.1038/s41393-017-0010-x

[11] Levine DN. Sherrington's the integrative action of the nervous system: A centennial appraisal. Journal of the Neurological Sciences. 2007;**253**(1-2):1-6. DOI: 10.1016/j.jns.2006.12.002

[12] McDonald JW, Sadowsky C. Spinal-cord injury. Lancet. 2002;**359**(9304):417-425. DOI: 10.1016/S0140-6736(02)07603-1

[13] Hiersemenzel LP, Curt A, Dietz V. From spinal shock to spasticity: Neuronal adaptations to a spinal cord injury. Neurology. 2000;**54**(8):1574-1582. DOI: 10.1212/wnl.54.8.1574

[14] Lohana AC, Neel S, Deepak V, Schauer M. Intrathecal iodinated contrast-induced transient spinal shock. BML Case Reports. 2020;**13**(12):e237610. DOI: 10.1136/bcr-2020-237610

[15] Guttmann L. Spinal shock and reflex behaviour in man. Paraplegia. 1970;**8**(2):100-116. DOI: 10.1038/sc.1970.19

[16] Landau WM, Clare MH. The plantar reflex in man, with special reference to some conditions where the extensor response is unexpectedly absent. Brain.

1959;**82**(3):321-355. DOI: 10.1093/brain/82.3.321

[17] Riddoch G. The reflex functions of the completely divided spinal cord in man, compared with those associated with less severe lesions. Brain. 1917;**40**(2-3):264-402. DOI: 10.1093/brain/40.2-3.264

[18] Burke RE. Sir Charles Sherrington's the integrative action of the nervous system: A centenary appreciation. Brain. 2007;**130**(Pt 4):887-894. DOI: 10.1093/brain/awm022

[19] Conti K, Yellapu V, Sweeney J, et al. Spinal Shock: Differentiation from Neurogenic Shock and Key Management Approaches. London: IntechOpen; 2020

[20] Taylor MP, Wrenn P, O'Donnell AD. Presentation of neurogenic shock within the emergency department. Emergency Medicine Journal. 2017;**34**(3):157-162. DOI: 10.1136/emermed-2016-205780

[21] Yue JK, Tsolinas RE, Burke JF, et al. Vasopressor support in managing acute spinal cord injury: Current knowledge. Journal of Neurosurgical Sciences. 2019;**63**(3):308-317. DOI: 10.23736/S0390-5616.17.04003-6

[22] DO AF DPM. Assessment and Treatment of Spinal Cord Injuries and Neurogenic Shock [Internet]. JEMS: EMS, Emergency Medical Services - Training, Paramedic, EMT News. 2014 [cited 2023 Apr 27]. Available from: https://www.jems.com/patient-care/assessment-and-treatment-spinal-cord-inj/

[23] Consortium for Spinal Cord M. Early acute management in adults with spinal cord injury: A clinical practice guideline for health-care professionals. The Journal of Spinal Cord Medicine. 2008;**31**(4):403-479. DOI: 10.1043/1079-0268-31.4.408

[24] Stevens RD, Bhardwaj A, Kirsch JR, Mirski MA. Critical care and perioperative management in traumatic spinal cord injury. Journal of Neurosurgical Anesthesiology. 2003;**15**(3):215-229. DOI: 10.1097/00008506-200307000-00009

[25] Bilello JF, Davis JW, Cunningham MA, Groom TF, Lemaster D, Sue LP. Cervical spinal cord injury and the need for cardiovascular intervention. Archives of Surgery. 2003;**138**(10):1127-1129. DOI: 10.1001/archsurg.138.10.1127

[26] Jackson AB, Groomes TE. Incidence of respiratory complications following spinal cord injury. Archives of Physical Medicine and Rehabilitation. 1994;**75**(3):270-275. DOI: 10.1016/0003-9993(94)90027-2

[27] Christensen PB, Wermuth L, Hinge HH, Bomers K. Clinical course and long-term prognosis of acute transverse myelopathy. Acta Neurologica Scandinavica. 1990;**81**(5):431-435. DOI: 10.1111/j.1600-0404.1990.tb00990.x

Chapter 4

Extracorporeal Blood Purification with the Oxiris Membrane in Septic Shock

Franco Turani and Sara Martini

Abstract

Septic shock with AKI is associated with a high mortality. We evaluated whether continuous renal replacement therapy (CRRT) using a membrane (oXiris) with adsorbing properties could improve cardio-renal response and modulate endotoxin and cytokine levels. 105 patients requiring CRRT for septic shock-AKI received CRRT with an oXiris filter. The main cardio-renal parameters, SOFA total score, SOFA organ score, endotoxin and cytokine levels were measured at baseline (T0) and 72 h after the start of CRRT (T1). Norepinephrine infusion rate, blood lactate levels, and thromboelastographic parameters were monitored. At T1, the renal function improved ($p < 0.01$) urinary output increased (p < 0,.01) with the cardiac response and the decrease of norepinephrine infusion. SOFA total decreased to 8.4 ± 3 from 12 ± 2 ($p < 0.001$). Endotoxin decreased also at T 1 ($p < 0.01$) with a reduction of Il 6 and procalcitonin. Lactate level ranged from 3.37 ± 3.2mto 1.67 ± 1.8 mmol/l ($p < 0.01$). CRRT with the oxiris filter improves the cardio renal response response in septic patients with AKI. This is associated with a modulation of endo-toxemia, of cytokines and the stability of the coagulation parameters.

Keywords: blood purification, AKI, septic shock, Oxiris membrane, citrate anticoagulation

1. Introduction

Sepsis and septic shock are one of the 10 causes of death worldwide, and the second cause in Intensive Care Unit. Moreover, in many septic patients (e.g., 40%), acute kidney injury rapidly develops, increasing the risk of mortality (from 50 to 80%) and the complications [1]. Despite the clinical importance of AKI during sepsis, many physiological aspects are not completely known, and its treatment is currently inadequate. Only recently, new studies have challenged the hemodynamic nature of AKI during sepsis, which may occur even if the renal blood flow (RBF) is maintained [2].

In the context of sepsis, considering as a dysfunctional immunological response, probably many pro-inflammatory mediators and endotoxin may interact with the kidney at different levels (tubular cells, mesangial cells, glomerular cells) and induce AKI [3]. The kidney itself may exacerbate this inflammatory response and cross talk with other organ (lung, heart) to induce a multiorgan failure [4]. This may occur also in the recent viremia Covid-19, in which an uncontrolled inflammatory response is described by many AA and septic shock with a multiorgan failure may ensue.

Extracorporeal blood purification, combining renal replacement therapy with the adsorption of many mediators, may be useful to modulate the septic immunological response and halt the renal cross talk with other organs.

Many devices are widely used, with different adsorbing capacity, but with inconclusive results [5].

The AN69-based oXiris membrane is modified with a positively charged charged polyimine ethylene layer capable of adsorbing negatively charged endotoxin molecules and IL6, IL10, and other mediators. Broman et al. have shown that Oxiris membrane may adsorb endotoxin and IL6 better than AN 69 st. in the first 24 h of treatment of patients with abdominal sepsis [6].

In this prospective study, we evaluated the changes of endotoxin during 76 h of CRRT in patients with different sources of sepsis. The changes of IL6, IL10, and procalcitonin are also studied, with the assessment of the coagulation in an attempt to confirm the effect of oXiris on endotoxin and other mediators in septic patients with AKI in a time period study longer than 24 h.

2. Methods

2.1 Study design

Non-interventional, observational, multicenter, prospective study.

2.2 Study cohort

The setting was a 11-bed secondary referral medical-surgical intensive care unit (ICU) at the Aurelia Hospital in Rome, Italy, and the 15-bed Cardiothoracic Intensive Care at the European Hospital in Rome. All patients were treated according to the normal ICU protocol and current severe sepsis guidelines [7].

The study population consisted of patients with sepsis/septic shock defined by Sepsis 3 conference with AKI, defined by KDIGO criteria. (Sepsis 3 Kdigo) Inclusion criteria were also considered: Endotoxin activity assay $\geq$0.6 and/or IL6 $\geq$ 150 pg/mL, noradrenaline infusion, MAP, and P/F ratio < 200 with mechanical ventilation or NIV. Patients with an age < 18 years 80 > and/or being pregnant, if present chronic renal failure (or previous treatment with CRRT), endotoxin or interleukins in the normal range, Glasgow Coma Score (GCS) < 8 due to hemorrhagic or ischemic events, and the need of extracorporeal membrane oxygenation (ECMO) were not eligible to receive CRRT and Oxiris treatment.

2.3 Study procedure

After receiving consent, Oxiris filter (Baxter, Il_USA) was assembled on the Prismaflex System or Prismamax (Il_USA), and CRRT was started on CVVHDF mode.

All treatments were performed by the same experienced nurses under the supervision of the investigators. Vascular access was obtained with use of double-lumen venous catheters through echographic visualization of femoral or Iinternal giugular vein. The circuit was prepared according to the manufacturer's guidelines

Qb ml/min	150 ± 20
Qd ml/h	1000 ± 600
Qr pre dilution ml/h	0
Qr post dilution ml/h	800 ± 250
Q PBP citrate infusion ml/h	1400 ± 250
Filtration fraction (%)	25 ± 6

Table 1.
CVVHDF with oXiris filter: initial prescription.

Anticoagulation	N. patients	Hours of treatment
Heparin ev	10	26 ± 5
Citrate 10 mmol/L	10	32 ± 8
Citrate 18 mmol/L	70	56 ± 16
No anticoagulation	11	18 ± 6

Table 2.
CVVHDF with oXiris filter: anticoagulation of the circuit.

by rinsing the device with 1000 ml of physiological saline solution with 5000 UI of heparin.

In **Tables 1** and **2**, the initial prescription of CRRT with oXiris membrane and the protocols of anticoagulation we used are shown.

2.4 Measurement

Endotoxin activity was measured using a commercial kit for whole blood neutrophil-dependent chemiluminescence (EAA Endotoxin Activity Assay; Spectral Diagnostics, Inc., Toronto, Ont., Canada). Arterial blood samples for EAA assay were drawn before the treatment (T0), after 72 h of CRRT with the Oxiris membrane (T1). The plasma levels of IL-6 and IL 10 were measured using enzyme-linked immunosorbent assay kits, according to the manufacturer's instructions (R&DSystems, Minneapolis, MN, USA). PCT was detected by enzyme-linked fluorescence assay (MINIVIDAS; bioMérieux, Marcy-l'Étoile, France).

Hemodynamic and respiratory data were continuously recorded on the electronic patient record system. Transthoracic echocardiography was performed by a cardiologist blind to the protocol, and the images was stored and analyzed off-line.

Thromboelastography analysis was performed at basal time and at the end of the treatment.

The Thrombelastograph® (TEG® 5000, Haemonetics Inc., Braintree MA) analyzer, the TEG6s system (Haemonetics, Braintree, MA, Niles, IL) have been used.

2.5 End points

Primary end points

1. Improvement of renal failure with the decrease of SOFA renal to 50% of the basal level

2. Increase of urinary output of 50% vs. basal level, improvement of the fluid balance, and increase of P/F ratio

3. Resolution of the arterial hypotension and decrease of the vasoactive drugs with the changes of SOFA cardio to 50% of the basal level

4. Decrease of SOFA total to 40% of the basal level

Secondary end points

1. Decrease of endotoxin to <0.6 and IL6 to 40% of the basal level

2. Decrease of procalcitonin and PAI-1 to 40% of the basal level

3. Stability of the coagulation profile, included thromboelastographic parameters and changes of PAI-1

4. Improvement of filter thrombogenicity, evaluated by Platelet map thromboelastography

2.6 Data collection

All clinical data are stored on the clinical informatic platform CLINIC DATA PRO (System Line—Empoli, Italy). All microbiological, immunological, and coagulation data are stored on the laboratory informatic platform—MODULAB GOLD ITALY (WERFEN UK). The data of 25 patients were transmitted and stored on the clinical platform REDCUP Villa.

2.7 Ethical consideration

The study protocol was approved by the Ethics Committee of the Azienda Ospedaliera San Camillo – Forlanini (reference No. 418 CE Lazio 1/2019) and registered at clinicaltrials.gov (NCT03914586). Written informed consent was obtained from each patient or next of kin.

2.8 Statistical analysis

Sample size calculation was based on changes in EAA level detected using the EAA test in a previous study on oXiris in patients with AKI and septic shock [BPUF]. Using a Student's paired t-test with a two-sided $\alpha = 0.05$, it was calculated that 90% power would be obtained with a sample size of 60 patients, based on a decrease in endotoxin levels from 0.78[0.98–0.65] EU/ to 0.58 [0.13–0.41] EU/ml. To compensate for potentially larger variation in endotoxin levels, we estimated that 80 patients with complete datasets should be included.

Continuous variables are reported as mean ± SD or median (first–third quartiles) and categorical variables as count and proportion. Comparisons of proportions were made using Chi-square test or Fisher exact test. Continuous variables were compared using Student t-test or Wilcoxon rank-sum test and one-way anal-ysis of variance or Kruskal-Wallis test, as appropriate. Post hoc Tukey range test and Dunn's test for multiple comparisons were used. We performed stepwise (forward and backward) multivariable logistic regression analyses to identify factors associated with different types of infections.

We performed multivariate analyses to identify factors potentially associated with different infections: abdominal infection vs. thoracic infection. Covariates found to be associated with abdominal infection in the bivariate analysis with a p value of less than or equal to 0.20 were entered in stepwise (forward and backward) multivariable logistic regression analyses with significance alpha levels less than or equal to 0.05 for retention. Multicollinearity was assessed calculating a variance inflation factor of each variable and rules out if the variance inflation factor was lower than 4. Results are shown as ORs with 95% CIs, and model performance was assessed using the Hosmer-Lemeshow goodness-of-fit test statistic. These analyses were conducted with GraphPad Prism 7.02 (La Jolla, CA, USA).

3. Results

From January 2012 to September 2020, 143 patients with sepsis septic shock (Sepsis III definition) and AKI (AKIN classification) required ICU admission to Aurelia Hospital and European Hospital in Rome.

Among these patients, after the revision of the clinical data stored in the clinical informatic platform, 42 patients have been excluded from the study, as they did not fulfill the inclusion criteria (**Figure 1**).

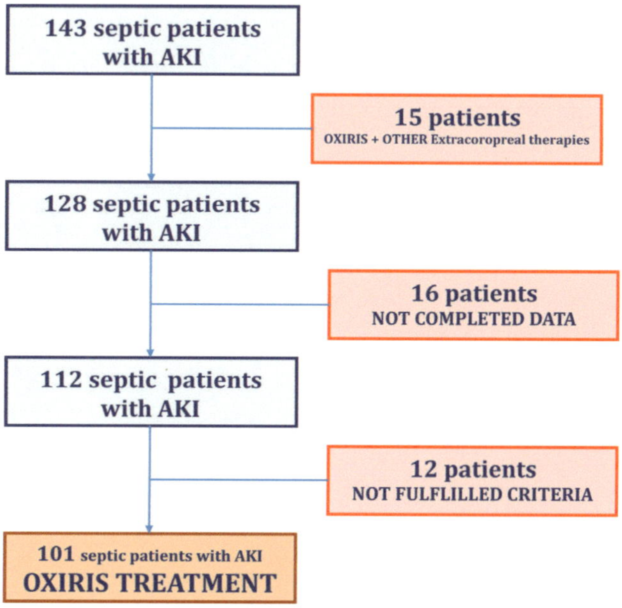

Figure 1.
Enrollment of the patients in the study. From 143 patient referred to the two intensive care AURELIA HOSPITAL and EUROPEAN HOSPITAL finally 101 patients were enrolled in the study.

In total, 101 patients with sepsis/septic shock and AKI (AKIN criteria) received CRRT with oXiris filter and completed the study. In **Tables 3** and **4**, the main basal anthropometric and clinical data are reported. All patients received intensive care treatment in accordance with the Survive Sepsis Campaign Bundle. The initial prescription was continuous venovenous hemodiafiltration (CVVHDF), as reported in **Table 1**. Data on anticoagulation are shown in **Table 2**.

For the 101 patients included in the study, we analyzed the protocol data at basal time (T0) and after 72 h of treatment (T1). All patients included in the study were also stratified on AKIN criteria, and the changes between these groups were also evaluated.

3.1 Primary end points

During the 72 h of treatment, urinary output increased and creatinine improved (**Table 5**). SOFA renal decreased (**Figure 2**). Urinary output increased to 57% and was associated with the increase of P/F ratio and fluid balance (**Tables 5** and **6**).

In **Table 6**, the main hemodynamic changes during the treatment are shown. MAP increased and norepinephrine dosage dropped to low value. This is associated with the changes of SOFA cardio.

SOFA total decreased, too, as a result of this global clinical improvement (**Figure 2**).

3.2 Secondary end points

At T0, EE activity was 0.64 ± 0.15. 8.5% of patients had low EAA activity (< *0.39 unit*), 28% medium EAA activity (*0.40–0.59 unit*), and 63% of patients high EAA activity (> *0.60 unit*), confirming the massive release of endotoxin in septic patients with AKI.

Number of patients	**101**
M/F	68/33
Age/year	68 ± 9
Weight (kg)	85 ± 15
Height (cm)	170 ± 6
BSA	2.2 ± 0.6

Table 3.
The main anthropometric data at study entry.

APACHE II	23 ± 4
SOFA total	12.6 ± 3
AKIN Classification	
AKI 3 patients	36
AKI 2 patients	27
AKI 1 patients	38

Table 4.
Basal clinical data at study entry.

	T0	T1
Creatinine mg/dl	2.3 ± 1	1.15 ± 0.5***
UOP mL/24 h	1074 ± 825	1826 ± 1173***
HCO3 meq/l	21 ± 2	24 ± 3
Lactate mmol/l	2.3 (1.6–3.2)	1.1 (0.8–1.8)**

**** $p < 0.001$*
*** $p < 0.01$*

Table 5.
Renal and metabolic changes during CRRT with the membrane oXiris.

	T0	T1
MAP mmHg	63 ± 12	79 ± 13***
Noradrenaline μicr/kg/min	0.12 ± 0.1	0.05 ± 0.01***
P/F ratio	215 ± 80	288 ± 73*
Arterial elastance	1.2 (1.1–1.4)	1.9 (1.3–2.05)
Ventricular elastance	0.7 (0.6–0.9)	1.2 (1.1–1.4)

**** $p < 0.001$*
*** $p < 0.01$*
** $p < 0.05$*

Table 6.
Hemodynamic and respiratory changes during CRRT with the membrane oXiris.

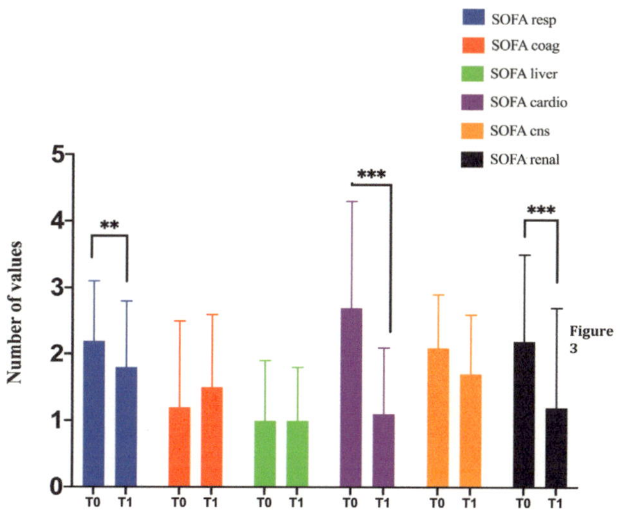

Figure 2.
SOFA changes during CRRT with oXiris filter. SOFA changes are shown. SOFA resp., SOFA card, SOFA renal improve. T0 = basal time. T1 = after 72 h of oXiris treatment.

At T1, EAA decreased to 0.5 ± 0.1 *unit* ($p < 0.01$ *vs T0*) Il6, Il 10, and procalcitonin mirrored these changes (**Table 7**).

	T0	T1
IL6 pg/ml	437 (206–1137)	91 (28–188)***
IL 10 pg/ml	14 (7–132)	8 (6–42)
Procalcitonin ng/ml	45 (14–58)	12 (10–18)***
EAA unit	0.64 ± 0.15	0.51 ± 0.1**

****** $p< 0.001$
**$p< 0.01$*

Table 7.
Immunological changes during CRRT with the membrane oXiris.

Parameters	T0	T1
Platelets (10^3 μl)	159 ± 124	127 ± 83
Fibrinogen (mg/dl)	507 ± 248	493 ± 248
D/dimer (ng/ml)	2402 ± 1136	2135 ± 1037
PAI-1 (ng/ml)	76 ± 31	25 ± 28*

*$p<0.05$.

Table 8.
Coagulation parameters during CRRT with oXiris filter.

Coagulation parameters were stable, with nonsignificant decrease of platelets and no changes of TEG parameters (**Table 8**).

PAI – I decreased, too, confirming an antithrombotic effect of RRT with oxiris membrane, as indicated by platelet TEG in patients with citrate anticoagulation.

3.3 Adverse events

Clotting of the filter (5/20) and minor bleeding (8/20) were the most common events in patients with heparine anticoagulation. Patients with citrate anticoagulation developed acid-base disturbance (metabolic acidosis 7/70, lactic acidosis 5/70), clotting of the filter (10/70), and two episodes of HIT not related completely to the CRRT treatment. In the patients treated without anticoagulation, clotting of the filter was a common event (6/11).

4. Discussion

4.1 Key findings

The main findings of this study are:

1. AKI during sepsis/septic shock is associated with a pro-inflammatory response (IL6, Procalcitonin, Endotoxin), it's equally present in all the AKIN groups and drives a multiorgan dysfunction.

2. CRRT with the adsorbing filter oXiris may improve this condition: its use has a positive effect either on the cardio-renal function and the immunological response.

3. Despite the involvement of the coagulation system during sepsis/septic shock, CRRT with the oXiris filter seems to prevent the worsening of the coagulation and DIC.

4. This effect may result from an antithrombotic of the oXiris filter, mainly when anticoagulation with citrate is used.

AKI is a severe complication of sepsis: it's a common finding in 40–50% of septic patients and correlates with a high mortality. However, no effective therapy is currently available, and recent studies challenged the notion that AKI during sepsis depends on renal perfusion and systemic hypotension. New evidences suggest that a dysregulated immunological and inflammatory response induces microcirculatory alterations not responding to the usual intensive care treatment.

Data of our study confirm these results: IL6 is high at basal levels and probably has a direct toxic on the kidney and induce a vasoplegic response, which is also detrimental for the renal function.

Shimatsu et al. found that high quartiles of IL6 increased the risk of anuria and AKI, whereas Payen et al. found that plasma cytokine's profile differed according to AKI severity [8].

In adjunct to IL6, we also evaluated procalcitonin and endotoxin: they were elevated in all the AKIN groups. Procalcitonin increases during bacterial infection and during sepsis, may induce a toxic effect on the kidney, and is associated, too, with AKI development and mortality in critically ill patients, in line with our results. Very recently, Ronco et al. have shown that a combination of [TIMP-2] Å ~ [IGFBP7] and PCT improved the predictive ability for AKI occurrence. Unfortunately, in our study we did not measure biomarkers and we cannot confirm these data [9].

Nevertheless, the serial measurements of cytokines and procalcitonin and the changes of the renal function reinforce the Ronco's hypothesis that there is an association between inflammation and AKI development.

Interestingly more than 80% of patients, in our study, had endotoxin ≥0.6 ng/mL, a cutoff value, which correlates with a predictive positive response to BP in Euphrates trial.

In our study, as in Euphrates RCT, we enrolled patients with different infections (GRA– and GRAM+) or none (**Table 9**). Endotoxiemia, therefore, seems a global response during sepsis and AKI, not depending only on Gram-negative infections, but also on Gram + bacteria and probably by bacterial translocation, as recently pointed out by Honore' et al. [10].

The IL10 changes follow the changes of all other mediators, confirming that a pro- and anti-inflammatory response may coexist in the early phase of the sepsis.

Pathogen	Number
Gram-negative	40
Gram-positive	20
Mixed gram negative and positive	25
No microbiological data	15
Fungi	5

Table 9.
Pathogens isolated in the study population.

This dysregulated immunological response translated in a multiorgan dysfunction with high basal lactate levels, the need of vasopressor therapy, and of mechanical ventilation in more than 80% of patients.

CRRT with Oxiris filter had many effects on this condition. First of all, this treatment improved the renal function: creatinine decreased and urinary output increased with improvement of SOFA renal (**Figure 1**). As expected, cardiocirculatory function improved: MAP increased with the decrease of noradrenaline infusion and SOFA cardiac (**Figure 1**).

These data are well explained in the context of the cardio-renal syndrome, in which oliguria, electrolytic disturbances, and uremia depress the cardiac function. However, the circulatory function during sepsis depends also on many inflammatory mediators. In this study, in effect, the improvement of the renal and the cardiac function is associated with the decrease of IL 6 and procalcitonin (**Table 7**).

Very recently, Zhay et al. showed a superiority of oxiris filter in confront of RRT with no adsorbing filter, with data on il6 endotoxin and cardio-renal response similar to our study. Notably, they showed also the changes of procalcitonin, as in our study. These data are recently confirmed by Xie et al., who stated that the changes of procalcitonin during the treatment may have a positive impact on the survival [9, 11, 12].

We observed also the changes of the endotoxin. This is in agreement with Kellum's in vitro study and Broman's and Zai's et al.'s clinical studies [7, 11].

Different from these studies, we used a chemiluminescence method to detect EAA changes during a longer time study. Whereas Broman and Zai evaluated EAA changes during 24- and 8-h treatment; in our study, EAA changes are evaluated at basal time and after 72 h of treatment.

Notably, endotoxin improved more in sepsis of abdominal origin then in thoraco-pulmonary sepsis, as previously shown by Cutuli et al. [13]. Probably in our study, as in Euphas 2, patients with abdominal infection have a more rapid decrease of endotoxin trough the source control of surgery. In this case, endotoxin declines rapidly also at extracellular and tissue level, promoting a more efficient adsorbing effect of the membrane **Figure 3**.

This important pro-inflammatory reaction, as expected, activates the coagulation response: platelets are in the lower normal range, PAI-1 is increased, and TEG analysis showed high or normal MA in more of 50% of patients, confirming that hypercogulation is a common trait during sepsis [14].

During the treatment, all coagulation parameters are stable or improve, as indicated by D/D, the stability of the platelet's numbers and decrease of PAI-1. Data of TEG, too, indicate a stability of all parameters.

We can hypothesize that some properties of the oXiris filter—heparine-coated layers, the adsorbing action of pro-inflammatory, and pro-coagulant mediators with the use of regional anticoagulation with citrate may modulate the coagulation cascade and prevent DIC.

However, heparin-coated membrane itself, as assembled on oXiris membrane, probably fails to prevent a full anticoagulation. Shetz et al., Seminars et al. reported that AN69 ST membrane and Oxiris membrane do not prolong filter survival without anticoagulation [15, 16].

Probably heparin-coated layers may be saturated very early, as the anticoagulant effect is likely localized to only areas of membranes where heparin is immobilized and exposed areas to politylenimine are not spared by thombogenicity.

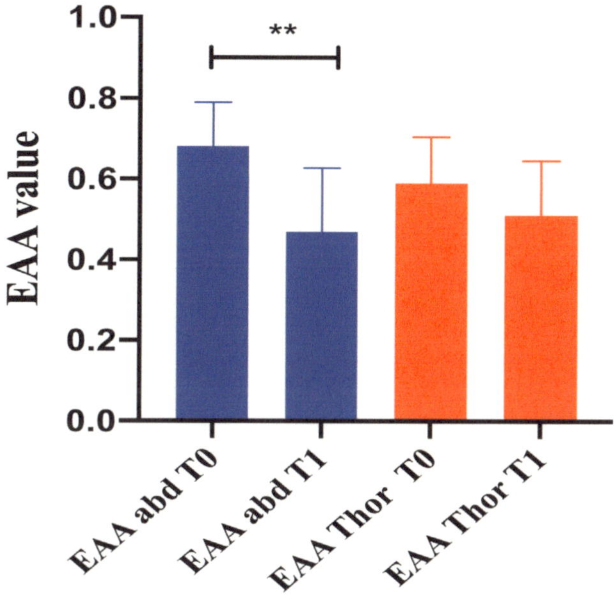

Figure 3.
Endotoxin response during CRRT with oXiris filter in different infection patients. In patients with sepsis of abdominal origin (abd) endotoxin decreases more than in patients with sepsis of thoracopulmonary (thor) origin. $^{**}p$ < 0.01 in the group.

Secondarily, during sepsis, activated monocite and other cells adhere to surface of extracorporeal circuit, inhibit fibrinolysis, and render clots resistant to heparin [17].

Third heparin has a weak activity on calcium concentration, whereas during sepsis, the most important pro-coagulant mechanism is induced by calcium release.

Finally, histones and other dams or pumps are strongly adsorbed by heparin layers, which may be early saturated and then inhibited to anticoagulate the membrane [18]. Thus, citrate protocol we used in this study seems a rational alternative to heparin [14].

The main advantage of citrate is that regional anticoagulation achieves optimal filter anticoagulation without affecting patient's coagulation. In this study, the coagulation parameters are stable, without induction of avert DIC.

In **Table 10**, the changes of TEG parameters during oXiris treatment are shown.

In **Figure 4**, the different changes of them during citrate and heparin anti coagulation are shown. In the heparin group MA and R were longer than citrate group, confirming that citrate achieves a better stability of the coagulation.

These data are in line with a very recent study by Osterman et al., who confirmed that coagulation profiles were stable during CRRT with citrate and no increase of prothrombotic status was found. Wiegele et al. confirmed these data [18].

We aimed, also, to control the in-filter changes of the coagulation to confirm whether citrate would be able to abolish the coagulation, as compared with heparin. Filter was fully anticoagulated by citrate, but not by heparin (**Figure 5**). This was little surprising, considering that heparin is widely used to anticoagulate all the extra corporeal circuits in many clinical contexts.

During sepsis, however, a pro-coagulant response is activated, either through calcium-dependent mechanism or inhibition of normal anticoagulant factors

Parameters	T0	T1
R (min)	9.65 ± 3	9.59 ± 4
K (min)	2.1 ± 0.5	3.7 ± 0.9
Ang (grade)	65 ± 7	62 ± 9
MA (mm)	65 ± 5	76 ± 59 ± 8
LY 30 (%)	3 ± 0.9	6.5 ± 0.9

Table 10.
TEG parameters during CRRT with oXiris filter.

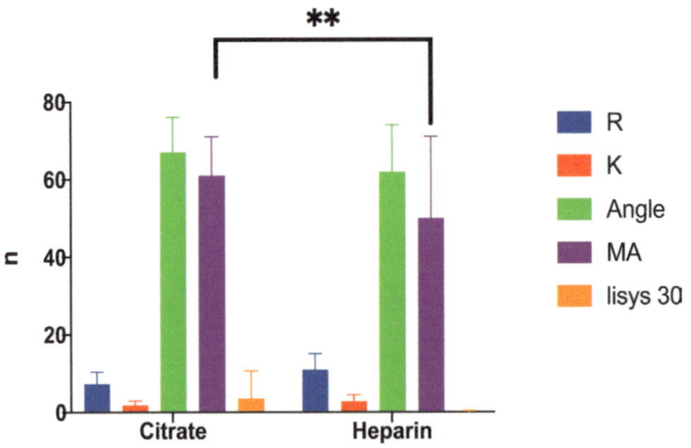

Figure 4.
*TEG changes during CRRT with oXiris filter from arterial sample. In citrate group, MA was higher than in heparin group, as a more firm coagulation is achieved ** p < 0.01 between the groups. R and K are expressed in min, ANG in grade, and MA in mm.*

(e.g., decrease of AT III). In this way, heparin response is blunted and thrombosis of circuits may occur, with failure of the treatments and worsening of the patient's condition [19].

These data are in line with Panigada et al., who reported that citrate infusion to maintain ca++ filter <0.25 mmol/L fullly anticoagulated the ECCO2 removal circuit and had TEG changes as in our study [20].

Ostermann et al., otherwise, have shown that citrate anticoagulation does not affect intra-circuit parameters and that all patients exhibited raised thrombin generation.

At variance with this study, we utilized the Haemonetic TEG, which employs a heparinized blood sample that is mixed with dried reagents within each of the four channels of the cartridge. We cannot hypothesize whether these different changes of TEG parameters depend on a different method, or reagents or a different properties of the dialytic membranes have been used.

Failure of the circuit depends not only on coagulation factors, by also on platelets, which are activated during sepsis and CRRT.

In this study, we evaluated also platelet's function by thromboelastography: this was downregulated in the filter during treatment with citrate, but not with heparin (**Figure 4**).

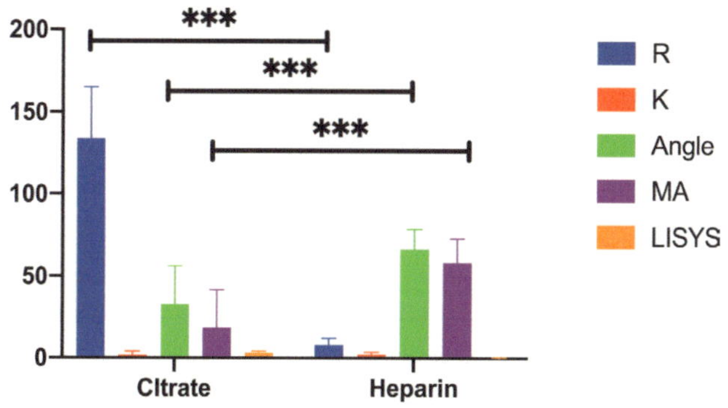

Figure 5.
*In filter changes during CRRT with oXiris filter. In citrate R was higher, angle and MA lower than heparin group, as a stronger filter anticoagulation. *** p < 0.001 between the groups. R and K are expressed in min, ANG in grade, and MA in mm.*

As platelets are activated via a calcium-dependent mechanisms, citrate probably decrease platelet activation in many ways, including inhibition of PF4, extracellulare vescicles, and particle microparticle, which are strongly pro-coagulant **Figure 5**.

Heparin, itself, may enhance platelet aggregation probably by P2Y receptor: the effect of Ca++ inhibition by and the action of heparin may explain the different TEG changes and confirm that citrate has a full anti coagulation, better than heparin [21].

These data are, again, at difference with Ostermann, who observed no change in platelets function, using PFA-100 analyzer. Panigada, too, did not show any effect of citrate on platelet function evaluated by aggregometry. Also in this case we can conclude whether these divergent data stem from different methods of study or from an effect of the oXiris membrane we used.

Conflict of interest

Dottor Franco Turani received a research grant by Baxter Healthcare, Chicago, USA.

Author details

Franco Turani[1,2]* and Sara Martini[1]

1 Intensive Care, Aurelia Hospital, Rome, Italy

2 Intensive Care, Cardiothoracic Surgery, European Hospital, Rome, Italy

*Address all correspondence to: turani.franco44@gmail.com

References

[1] Lameire NH, Bagga A, Cruz D, De Maeseneer J, Endre Z, Kellum JA, et al. Acute kidney injury: An increasing global concern. Lancet. 2013;**382**:170-179. DOI: 10.1016/S0140-6736(13)60647

[2] Maiden MJ, Otto S, Brealey JK, Finnis ME, Chapman MJ, Kuchel TR, et al. Structure and function of the kidney in septic shock. A prospective controlled experimental study. American Journal of Respiratory and Critical Care Medicine. 2016;**194**:692-700. DOI: 10.1164/rccm.201511-2285OC

[3] Bellomo R, Kellum JA, Ronco C, Wald R, Martensson J, Maiden M, et al. Acute kidney injury in sepsis. Intensive Care Medicine. 2017;**43**:816-828. DOI: 10.1007/s00134-017-4755-7

[4] Dellepiane S, Marengo M, Cantaluppi V. Detrimental cross-talk between sepsis and acute kidney injury: New pathogenic mechanismsearly biomarkers and targeted therapies. Critical Care. 2016;**20**:61. DOI: 10.1186/s13054-016-1219-3

[5] Supady A, Brodie D. Tobias Wengenmayer Extracorporeal haemoadsorption: Does the evidence support its routine use in critical care? The Lancet Respiratory Medicine. 2022;**10**:307-312

[6] Broman ME, Hansson F, Vincent JL, Bodelsson M. Endotoxin and cytokine reducing properties of the oXiris membrane in patients with septic shock: A randomized crossover double-blind study. PLoS One. 2019;**14**:e0220444

[7] Surviving Sepsis Campaign. International guidelines for management of severe sepsis and septic shock: Intensive Care Medicine. 2008;**34**:17-60. DOI: 10.1007/s00134-007-0934-2

[8] Payen D, Lukaszewicz A-C, Legrand M, Gayat E, Faivre V, et al. A multicentre study of acute kidney injury in severe sepsis and septic shock: Association with inflammatory phenotype and HLA genotype. PLoS One. 2012;**7**(6):e35838. DOI: 10.1371/journal.pone.0035

[9] Godi et al. Urinary [TIMP-2] Å~ [IGFBP7] and serum procalcitonin to predict and assess the risk for short-term outcomes in septic and non-septic critically ill patients. Annals of Intensive Care. 2020;**10**:46

[10] Honore P et al. Efficacy of polymyxin B hemoperfusion in and beyond septic shock: Is an "endotoxinseverity score" needed? Critical Care. 2018;**22**:205. DOI: 10.1186/s13054-018-2093-y

[11] Zhai J et al. The application value of oXiris-endotoxin adsorption in sepsis. American Journal of Translational Research. 2021;**13**(4):3839-3844

[12] Xiao X. Effect of oXiris-CVVH on the clinical outcomes of patients with septic shock: An inverse probability of treatment-weighted analysis. Blood Purification:3, 1-18. DOI: 10.1159/000524088

[13] Cutuli et al. Polymyxin-B hemoperfusion in septicpatients: Analysis of a multicenter registry. Annals of Intensive Care. 2016;**6**:77

[14] Fisher et al. Effects of regional citrate anti coagulation on thrombin generation, fibrinolysis and platelet function in critically ill patients receiving continuous renal replacement therapy for acute kidney injury: A prospective study. Annals of Intensive Care. 2022;**12**:29. DOI: 10.1186/s13613-022-01004

[15] Schetz M et al. Does the surface-treated AN69 membraneprolong filter survival in CRRT without anticoagulation? Intensive Care Medicine. 2012;**38**:1818-1825

[16] Wong EY, Ong V, Remani D, et al. Filter life and safety of heparin-grafted membrane forcontinuous renal replacement therapy—A randomizedcontrolled trial. Seminars in Dialysis. 2021;**00**:1-9

[17] Semeraro F, Ammollo CT, Semeraro N, Colucci M. Tissue factor-expressingmonocytes inhibit fibrinolysis through a TAFI-mediated mechanism, and make clots resistant to heparins. Haematologica. 2009;**94**:819-826. DOI: 10.3324/haematol.2008.000042

[18] Heparin-Functionalized Adsorbents Eliminate Central Effectors of Immunothrombosis, including Platelet Factor 4, High-Mobility Group Box 1 Protein and Histones. International Journal of Molecular Sciences. 1823;**2022**:23. DOI: 10.3390/ijms23031823

[19] Thrombin provokes degranulation of platelet α-granules leading to the release of active plasminogen activator inhibitor-1 (PAI-1). Shock. 2018;**50**(6):671-676

[20] Scaravilli V et al. Effects of sodium citrate, citric acid and lactic acid on human blood coagulation. Perfusion. 2018;**33**(7):577-583

[21] Wiegele M, Infanger L, Lacom C, Koch S, Baierl A, Schaden E. Thrombin generation and platelet function in ICU patients undergoing CVVHD using regional citrate anticoagulation. Frontiers in Medicine. 2021;**8**:680540. DOI: 10.3389/fmed.2021.680540

Chapter 5

Overview of Venoarterial Extracorporeal Membrane Oxygenation (VA-ECMO) Support for the Management of Cardiac Arrest and Cardiogenic Shock

Pankaj Garg, John H. Yazji, Emad Alamouti-Fard, Ishaq Wadiwala, Mohammad Alomari, Md Walid Akram Hussain, Mohamed Samir Hassan Elawady, Saqib Masroor and Samuel Jacob

Abstract

In the United States, ~100,000 patients are hospitalized annually for cardiogenic shock with 27–51% mortality. Similarly, ~356,000 patients develop out-of-hospital cardiac arrests (OHCA) annually with 90% mortality. In the last few decades, several acute mechanical circulatory support (AMCS) devices have been developed to provide hemodynamic support and to improve outcomes in patients with cardiogenic shock and cardiac arrest. Among all the devices, venoarterial extracorporeal membrane oxygenation (VA-ECMO) is the only AMCS device that provides immediate and complete cardiopulmonary support. With an increase in clinical experience with VA-ECMO, use of VA-ECMO has expanded beyond post-cardiotomy cardiogenic shock. In the last two decades, there has also been a rapid growth in the observational and randomized data describing the clinical and logistical considerations with successful clinical outcomes in patients with cardiogenic shock and cardiac arrest. In this review, we discuss the fundamental concepts and hemodynamic aspects of VA-ECMO, its indications, contra-indications, and the complications that are encountered in the setting of VA-ECMO in patients with cardiac arrest and cardiogenic shock of various etiologies.

Keywords: cardiogenic shock, cardiac arrest, ECPR, extracorporeal membrane oxygenation, myocardial infarction, sepsis, heart failure

1. Introduction

Extra corporeal membrane oxygenator (ECMO) is a type of cardiopulmonary life support in which blood is withdrawn from the venous system, circulated outside the body by a mechanical pump, and oxygenated carbon dioxide is removed with the help of a membrane oxygenator and then pumped back into the arterial (VA-ECMO) or venous system [1, 2]. ECMO provides an opportunity for both heart and lungs to rest and recover while body perfusion is maintained. Also, it helps to prolong the lives of patients on the waitlist for transplants list [3].

The history of ECMO dates back to 1944 when Kloff et al. were able to oxygenate blood when it was passed through the chambers of their artificial kidney [4]. Nine years after this breakthrough accomplishment, it was clinically applied when John Gibbon in 1953 repaired an atrial septal defect in an 18-year-old female on cardiopulmonary bypass (CPB) [5, 6]. After the introduction of Mayo-Gibbon machine in 1955, oxygenator becomes an integral part of CPB machine used for repairing cardiac defects [7]. In 1972, CPB machine was used for the first time for prolonged cardiopulmonary support for shock lung in a 24-year trauma patient with tear in thoracic aorta and other orthopedic injuries. The patient was supported on CPB machine for 75 hours and subsequently recovered [8]. Other cases quickly followed where CPB was used for prolonged cardiopulmonary support called extracorporeal life support (ECLS) [9, 10]. However, consistently poor outcomes in the majority of patients led to abandonment of ECMO. In 1976, Robert Bartlett used ECMO on a neonate suffering from meconium aspiration pneumonitis as rescue therapy. The baby recovered after 3 days and was successfully weaned from ECMO. This also led to the revival of ECMO to use as ECLS [11]. Earlier ECMO circuits had many problems including large circuits, large priming volume, the presence of bladder reservoir that increased the risk of air embolism, and roller pump that increased the risk of hemolysis, air, and particle embolism. Further, earlier ECMO was highly labor-intensive requiring constant vigilance to prevent the accidents. The ECMO circuit was initially optimized by Ken Litzie in 1983 decreasing the parts and intricacy of the machine, allowing for rapid deployment in a nonhospital setting [12]. With further improvement in machine design, use of centrifugal flow pumps with magnetically levitated rotating heads and use of silicone membrane oxygenators have made ECMO circuit low profile and less labor-intensive, and support the patient on ECMO safely for days to weeks without major complications. Although the origin of both CPB and ECMO machines is from same root, there are significant differences between both as summarized in **Table 1** [13].

Despite significant improvement in the ECMO circuit design, until 2009, ECMO was frequently used only for pediatric patients with good outcome. However, use of veno-venous ECMO (VV-ECMO) during the swine flu pandemic in 2009 with good outcome led to the revival of ECMO in adults. This was further boosted by successful use of ECMO in patients with COVID pneumonia during recent pandemic. Presently, ECMO circuit can be easily transported in both air and ground ambulances and instituted in a variety of cardiac and noncardiac conditions at various facilities like in the ward, operating room, cath lab, and even in the fields (mobile ECMO programs) at the site of cardiac arrest (CA) and even with ongoing cardiopulmonary resuscitation (CPR). Further, ECMO can provide robust biventricular as well as respiratory support in patients with severe refractory CS for prolonged duration with a patient being extubated and ambulant. Full VA-ECMO support offers time to perform diagnostic and therapeutic interventions while maintaining appropriate hemodynamics and gas exchange and organ perfusion.

In this chapter, we will review basics of ECMO and various indications of ECMO in patients with cardiogenic shock (CS) and cardiac arrest.

	ECMO	CPB
Pump	Centrifugal	Roller
Heparinization	50–100 units/kg	200–300 units/kg
Circuit type	Open	Closed
Maximal duration of circulation	Weeks	Hours
Ischemia of lower limbs	Common (peripheral ECMO)	Rare
Bleeding complications	Less frequent	More frequent
Activated clotting time (ACT) necessary	150–170 s	>400 s
Reservoir	Absent	Present
Open air contact	Absent	Present

Table 1.
Comparison of ECMO and CPB.

1.1 Components

ECMO circuit consists of venous and arterial cannulas for drainage and return of blood, respectively, a hollow fiber membrane oxygenator for blood oxygenation and carbon dioxide (CO2) clearance, and a centrifugal pump for propelling the blood. The presence of membrane oxygenator is a critical distinguishing feature of ECMO from other acute mechanical circulatory support (AMCS) devices.

1.2 Cannulation technique

ECMO can be placed centrally or peripherally. Central VA-ECMO is usually placed in post-cardiotomy setting, when venous drainage cannula is placed in the right atrium (RA) or superior vena cava (SVC) and inferior vena cava (IVC) separately and oxygenated blood is returned directly into the ascending aorta. For the management of CS, peripheral VA-ECMO is most commonly performed and femoral artery (FA), and femoral vein (FV) is the most commonly cannulated. Alternate site of cannulation is axillary artery or subclavian artery for arterial return and internal jugular vein (IJV) for venous drainage. Artery can be cannulated percutaneously under fluoroscopic guidance or surgically with a chimney graft. The advantages of whole upper body cannulation are ambulation, lower risk of infection, limb ischemia, cannula site bleeding, and ease of maintaining sterility. However, more time-consuming needs the presence of a surgeon. On the other hand, femoral cannulation can be easily done percutaneously by an individual trained in ECMO cannulation and is rapid. Appropriate size cannula should be selected to reduce the risk of vascular injury and at the same time maintain the low negative inflow (preferably <−50 mmHg) and low outflow (<300 mmHg) pressures [14]. In our center, when femoral artery is cannulated for VA-ECMO, we always insert a 6 Fr distal reperfusion cannula into the superficial femoral artery to mitigate the risk of distal limb ischemia and splice into the arterial limb of the circuit (**Figure 1**).

1.3 Hemodynamic aspects of VA-ECMO support

Among all the available AMCS devices, VA-ECMO has the highest capability to reduce myocardial pressure-volume area (sum of myocardial potential energy and

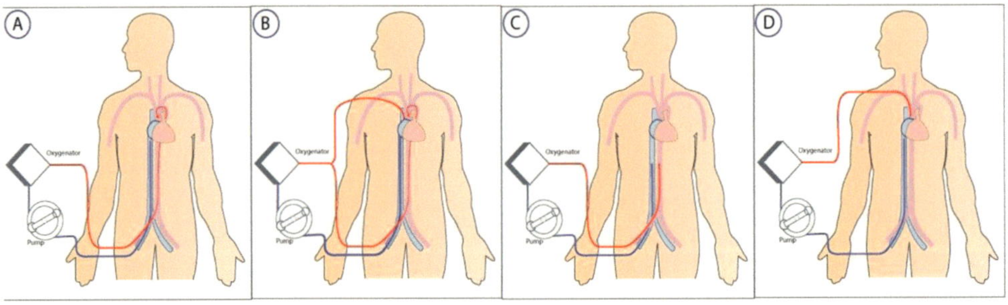

Figure 1.
Various cannulation sites for venoarterial extracorporeal membrane oxygenator.

myocardial stroke work) in patients with CS reducing left ventricular end-diastolic volume (LVEDV) and left ventricular end-diastolic pressure (LVEDP) while providing complete hemodynamic and respiratory support. Myocardial pressure-volume area is further reduced by the weaning of inotropes and vasopressors. All these prevent the vicious cycle of maladaptive neurohormonal and vascular mechanisms. Also, native RV function is not critical to provide systemic perfusion due to its reduced reliance on transpulmonary flow.

VA-ECMO improves systemic perfusion by increasing the MAP, reducing CVP, and increasing the systemic arteriovenous pressure gradient. This maintains the organ function and reduces the generation and accumulation of toxic metabolites. This may be particularly relevant to improving blood flow in organs with portal circulation, such as the liver and kidney. Fluid removal and reducing the venous congestion can be further enhanced by splicing a continuous veno-venous hemodialysis machine (CVVHD) into the VA-ECMO circuit [15–19].

1.4 LV distension

The Achilles heel of VA-ECMO is LV distension. The LV distension occurs when LV is unable to eject the blood returning to it. Sources for blood return to the LV are aortic regurgitation, Thebesian and bronchial veins draining in the left atrium, and systemic venous return that is not captured by the ECMO venous cannula. Uncaptured systemic venous return is the most significant source of LV blood flow, and it is directly proportional to RV function. Due to the lack of reservoir and longer and thinner peripheral venous cannulas with higher impedance, a significant amount of blood escapes drainage. To eject the blood, LV must have enough contractile function to overcome afterload due to retrograde flow of blood toward aortic valve at a higher pressure. If LV is severely dysfunctional, it may be unable to generate enough pressure and aortic valve may remain closed throughout cardiac cycle. This leads to increased LV wall stress, and myocardial oxygen demands as well as the stasis of blood in the aortic root with a potential risk of thrombus formation. Also, elevated LVEDP may result in pulmonary edema, pulmonary hemorrhage, systemic, cerebral, and myocardial hypoxia. The risk of LV and aortic thrombus formation is higher with peripheral cannulation due to a larger column of aortic root blood stasis and carries the risk of embolization down the coronary arteries, head vessels, or body. Therefore, it is important to vent the LV during VA-ECMO in patients with noncompliant LV and a competent mitral valve [20].

1.5 Diagnosis

In a patient on VA-ECMO, a dilated and hypocontractile LV with or without severe MR, stagnation of blood on echocardiography, pulmonary artery diastolic pressure >25 mmHg, and an elevated PCWP on Swan-Ganz catheter monitoring are sufficient to diagnose LV distension [19].

1.6 Indications for LV venting and unloading

On ECMO, indicators of good LV decompression are AV opening with every beat, systemic arterial pulse pressure >10 mmHg, and low PCWP. As the initial therapy inotropes, vasopressors, diuretics, and CVVHD to aid with managing volume status should be tried. Additionally, ECMO flows should be titrated to the lowest acceptable level to reduce the LV afterload. If medical management fails, one should consider LV venting [21].

Percutaneous transvenous atrial septostomy can be created under fluoroscopic and echocardiographic guidance in the catheterization lab to vent the LV. However, LV decompression through atrial septostomy is limited and dependent upon associated MR.

1.7 Percutaneous devices for LV unloading

LV can be unloaded by percutaneous devices like intra-aortic balloon pump (IABP) Impella, and TandemHeart. Impella is more robust device for LV unloading, and it also improves systemic perfusion. Impella is particularly important in patients with severely reduced LV contractility [22]. In our institute, we institute both arterial cannula and Impella 5.5 through AxA over Y chimney graft and venous cannula through IJV. Advantages of our technique are ambulation and weaning and ECMO decannulation with oversewing the Y limb of the graft can be done under local anesthesia and sedation.

1.8 Open surgical and minimally invasive LV unloading

LV unloading can be done by a surgically placed vent into the LV *via* the right superior pulmonary vein or *via* LV apex. In nonpost-cardiotomy patients, a surgical vent can still be placed into the LV apex *via* a left anterolateral thoracotomy and sliced into the venous limb of the ECMO cannula. Compared to ECpella, this approach perfuses the oxygenated blood into the aortic root, brain, and upper body and it unloads both the RV and LV more efficiently [19, 23].

In a patient with VA-ECMO with LV venting, patient must have a right radial arterial line for oxygenation monitoring, and a Swan-Ganz catheter in place to check mixed venous saturation, PCWP, and PAP. Daily chest X-rays should be obtained to assess degree of pulmonary edema, Impella position, and ECMO venous cannula position. Echocardiography should be performed to ensure the Impella position and LV decompression [19].

1.9 Results

Studies by Patel et al., Tepper et al., and Pappalardo et al. have shown improved survival in patients supported with ECpella with reduced all cause 30-day mortality compared to patients supported with VA-ECMO with inotropes or surgical LV venting. The studies attributed this improved survival to Impella as Impella was an effective means of LV unloading and prevented worsened pulmonary edema. Furthermore, the ECpella patients had a higher rate of successful bridging to either further recovery or further therapy [24–26].

1.10 Complications of VA-ECMO

Major complications are bleeding and thromboembolism (**Figure 2**).

1.10.1 Bleeding

Bleeding occurs in 30–50% of patients on VA-ECMO primarily due to anticoagulation and platelet dysfunction. Bleeding may occur at the cannulation site or into the body cavities (e.g., brain, abdomen, pleural and pericardial space) and may require surgical exploration to achieve hemostasis

1.10.2 Thrombosis and thromboembolism

Systemic thromboembolism may occur due to thrombus formation in the arterial side of VA-ECMO circuit and has devastating consequences. Venous thrombosis may develop at the cannulation site with the development of deep venous thrombosis and pulmonary embolism. Arterial thrombosis may lead to limb ischemia and gangrene. To prevent complications, circuit should be regularly inspected for signs of clot

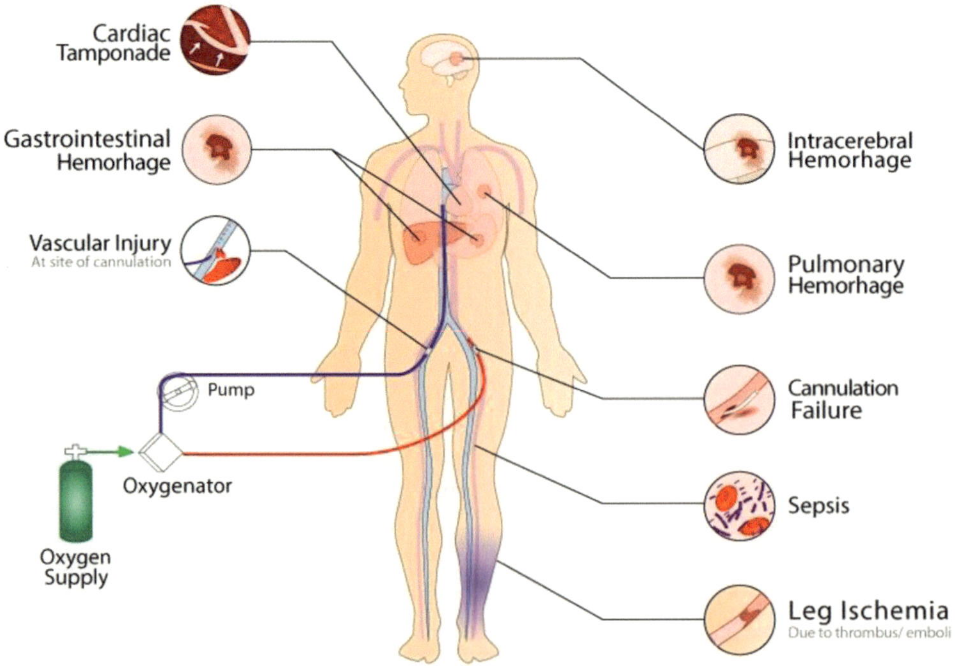

Figure 2.
Complications of VA-ECMO.

formation at the connectors site, tubing, and oxygenator, and monitoring the pressure gradient across the oxygenator. A sudden change in the pressure gradient suggests the development of thrombus. Large or mobile clots require immediate circuit or component exchange.

1.10.3 Neurological

The incidence of neurologic injury varies from 10% in adult respiratory failure patients to 50% in patients with ECPR. The types of neurological injury included coma, encephalopathy, anoxic brain injury, stroke, brain death, and myoclonus.

1.10.4 Cannulation-related

These complications are uncommon (<5%) and include vessel perforation with hemorrhage, arterial dissection, distal ischemia, and incorrect location (e.g., venous cannula within the artery).

1.10.5 Heparin-induced thrombocytopenia

Heparin-induced thrombocytopenia (HIT) can occur in patients receiving ECMO. When HIT is proven, the heparin infusion should be replaced by a nonheparin anticoagulant. We favor switching to bivalirudin in our institute.

1.11 VA ECMO-specific complications

- Pulmonary edema and hemorrhage, aortic root, and LV thrombus occur in patients who develop LV distension and stasis of blood in the LV and aortic root during VA ECMO. It is treated by venting the LA or LV.

- Coronary or cerebral hypoxia: Patients with good ventricular function and associated pulmonary pathology may develop coronary and cerebral hypoxia due to selective perfusion of the heart, brain, and upper extremities by LV blood. Condition is managed by infusing oxygenated blood into the right atrium (called VA-V ECMO).

1.12 Contraindication to VA-ECMO

For severe PAD (percutaneous only) and moderate or severe aortic regurgitation, although ECMO provides the highest level of support, it can lead to significant complications including pump thrombosis, bleeding, ischemic limbs, and Harlequin syndrome.

2. ECMO in cardiac arrest

Cardiac arrest is defined as the sudden cessation of cardiac activity as the victim is unresponsive, has no circulation, and is unable to breathe. The sudden cessation of cardiac activity may result in the death of the victim if not identified and treated quickly. It is a major public health hazard that impacts an estimated 356,500 people out of hospital and 209,000 people in the hospitals each year. An acute coronary syndrome is the most common cause of CA. Other common causes include pulmonary embolism, dyskalemia, acute respiratory failure, hypovolemia, sepsis, and poisoning [27]. Cardiac arrest can occur in hospital (IHCA) or outside hospital (OHCA). In a person with OHCA, cardiopulmonary resuscitation (CPR) should be initiated immediately. Mass public awareness, basic life support (BLS) training for general population, widespread availability of defibrillators, rapid response paramedic teams, and in-hospital CPR response teams, development of protocols for effective CPR have led to early and effective institution of CPR in patients with both OHCA and IHCA, especially in the developed countries; however, outcome remains dismal with <10% survival. The most important reason for high mortality after CA is the prolonged absence of blood flow to the brain and other vital organs leading to anoxic brain injury and irreversible damage to the other organs.

Till two decades back, conventional CPR (CCPR) including both basic life support and advanced cardiac life support (ACLS) was the best treatment plan for patient with CA as it would give them the best chance of survival. The purpose of doing CCPR in a patient with CA is to maintain the cerebral and coronary perfusion till the heart recovers its rhythm and contractility as the absence of cerebral blood flow for more than 3–5 minutes results in severe irreversible anoxic brain injury [28]. Studies have shown that despite effective CCPR, cerebral blood flow is only 30–40% of the resting blood flows [29]. Also, cardiac recovery with CCPR remains poor as it is unable to unload the distended LV. The distension of the heart after CA results in stretching of myofibrils beyond the physiological Frank-Starling limits. The myocardial stretching not only results in myocardial stunning but also myofibrils are unable to return to their normal resting tone unless the ventricle is empty. Therefore, despite effective BLS and ACLS, 30-day survival for a patient with OHCA is only 8–10.7%, while for IHCA the survival rate is 17–28% [30–32]. This high mortality rate led to develop new ways to treat people with CA. One of the techniques that have been developed is combining CPR with ECMO, which is known as extracorporeal cardiopulmonary resuscitation (ECPR) [33].

After the publication of few case reports about the successful use of ECMO in patients with in-hospital CA in 2008, there was renewed interest in use of ECMO in patients with out-of-hospital cardiac arrest (OHCA). Still, the use of ECMO on patients with OHCA in the United States is scarce (0.69% patients in 2014) with variable but encouraging survival (6–56%) [34–37]. A systematic review of 25 studies including patients with OHCA and IHCA showed quite variable and inconsistent outcomes with the use of ECPR. However, results of ECPR were consistently better in IHCA. This is due to difficulty in initiation of ECMO in the field. Therefore, patients with OHCA should be rapidly transported to the hospital and during transport, an automated external defibrillator (AED) should be used for automated cardioversion. Once patients arrive at the hospital, AED should be removed and ECMO is placed and initiated. Further study is needed to determine the effectiveness of the process and the survival rate [38].

3. Extracorporeal cardiopulmonary resuscitation

Extracorporeal cardiopulmonary resuscitation is an alternative method of providing cardiopulmonary resuscitation by using the ECMO device combined with CCPR in patients with CA and CS [39, 40]. ECMO takes over the function of the heart and lungs, and maintains the organ perfusion while allowing the time for heart and lung to recover and buy some time to investigate the cause of acute deterioration, to assess and treat underlying pathology to prolong the survival while minimizing complications. However, ECPR is a complex labor-intensive intervention that requires a highly trained team, specialized equipment, and multidisciplinary support within a healthcare system, and it has the risk of life-threatening complications including vessel rupture, bleeding, and thromboembolism. Therefore, physicians should carefully select patients for ECPR who can gain the most benefit, instead of applying ECPR indiscriminately.

4. Patient selection for ECPR

ECPR is a final effort employed in a patient with a deep circulatory shock after CA that is refractory to all standard treatments, and no further intervention will assuredly lead to the patient's demise. ECMO is brought in this scenario to assist with shock state while dithering to elucidate the cause of CA and later allows reversal if possible [41]. The American heart association guidelines advised that ECPR should be instituted in a patient if ECMO is rapidly available and deployable within a facility, patient has a brief duration from collapse, and the underlying condition is reversible [42]. As ECPR is a complex technique that requires an experienced and well-trained paramedic team, careful precision, teamwork, and coordinated efforts of a lot of persons to institute ECMO with ongoing, patients with CA should be carefully selected who can potentially benefit from ECPR [43].

In patient with OHCA, prognostic factors associated with better survival and neurological outcome are patient age <70 years, shorter duration of low flow, a sustained shockable rhythm, effective CPR with a target end-tidal carbon dioxide (EtCO2) > 10 mmHg during resuscitation, lower lactate level, higher pH, and lower SOFA score [44]. While these all criteria increase the likelihood of a favorable outcome, there are no universal selection criteria. Although there are no clearly defined indications, most

Positive	Negative
Age < 75 years old	Age > 75 years old
Initial shockable rhythm Pulseless VT/VF CA due to or resulting in VF	Non shockable rhythm
No ROSC within 15 mins of ACLS	CPR > 20 mins when the heart is in asystole (exceptions: hypothermia, drowning, and suspected pulmonary embolism) or VF/VT with ≥120 beats/min
CA due to reversible causes	CA due to Trauma or unamenable cause
High-quality CPR (ETCO2 ≥10 mm Hg)	Low-quality CPR (ETCO2 <10 mm Hg) Severely acidosis (pH < 6.8) or elevated lactate (≥20 mmol/L) Irreversible brain damage or poor neurological prognosis Severe comorbidity that would prevent independent life DNR/DNI or no consent given

VT = ventricular tachycardia, VF = ventricular fibrillation, ROSC = return of spontaneous circulation, DNR/DNI = do not resuscitate or intubate, CA = cardiac arrest, ETCO2 = end tidal carbon dioxide.

Table 2.
Positive and negative predictors of ECPR.

centers perform ECPR for young patients with an initial shockable rhythm or presumed correctable cause and those with a witnessed collapse and bystander CPR without ROSC within 10–20 minutes of CCPR. In patients with IHCA, ECPR is useful in patients with CA in the cardiac surgical ICU, medical cardiac ICU, cardiac catheterization laboratory, and CA before or after cardiac surgery or intervention. When a cardiac diagnosis is irreversible pathology, cardiac replacement therapy, such as heart transplantation or artificial heart, should be considered [45, 46]. Poor prognostic factors after ECPR are patients with poor physical activity levels such as those confined to bed; severe permanent neurologic injury; noncardiopulmonary cause of arrest, such as severe sepsis; prolonged CCPR without ROSC; inadequate ACLS, such as failed advanced airway or ineffective chest compression due to severe hypovolemia or unfavorable chest wall anatomy (e.g., aortic rupture or severe pectus excavatum); and pre-existing severe multiple organ failure. However, no single one can be considered an absolute contraindication for ECPR; the physician in charge of a patient's care should discuss resuscitation with leaders of the CPR and ECLS teams if the situation arises. Prognostic factors can be broken down into positive/negative factors influencing outcomes explained in **Table 2** [46].

5. Implementation of ECPR

Institution of ECMO in adult patient with CA is challenging and should be performed by an expert specialized in percutaneous ECMO cannulation [47, 48]. Cannulation can be done in various locations including femoral vessel, internal Jugular vein (IJV)-femoral artery, femoral vein-subclavian artery, or IJV-subclavian artery [49]. The femoral vessels are most common and most appropriate for cannulation as it is easiest to locate the femoral vessels blindly with the pulse guidance, under Doppler ultrasound guidance as well as surgically even in the absence of pulse and also with ongoing CPR as groins are away from site of resuscitation and more

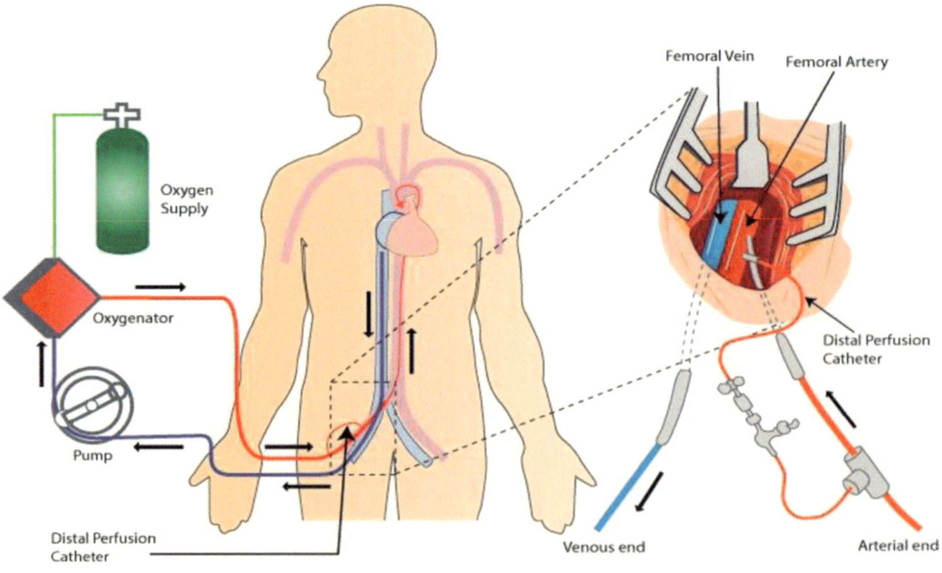

Figure 3.
Cannulation technique in ECPR.

space is available to work compared to subclavian artery and axillary arteries that are very close to the site of CPR and always crowded. Percutaneous technique is easier and quicker and does not require surgical skills. However, percutaneous technique is fraught with the risk of inability to puncture or cannulate the vessel [50]. With open surgical cannulation, it is easier to locate and cannulate the vessel of interest, but it significantly impacts procedure time [51]. Further, availability of cardiac or vascular surgeons for the exposure of femoral vessels and need for appropriate setup and instruments are additional hurdles for open surgical cannulation. Although, in pediatric patients with ECPR, open surgical cannulation of carotid artery and internal Jugular vein is the standard of care, in adults with CA, percutaneous cannulation of femoral vessels is preferred as time is the essence. But, if this fails, then an open surgical technique must be used [52]. In ECPR, selection of appropriate size cannulas is especially important as the size of cannula determines how efficiently the ECPR will work. The largest possible venous and arterial cannula appropriate to provide >2.5 L/m^2 flow with injuring the vessels should be selected. For an adult patient, 23–25 Fr venous drainage cannula and 17–19 Fr. arterial cannula are sufficient for adequate flow [41, 53]. The venous cannula is extended up to the right atrium or inferior vena cava and right atrial junction, and the arterial cannula is brought to the descending thoracic aorta (**Figure 3**).

6. Steps of institution of ECPR

With continued CPR, femoral artery and vein are cannulated percutaneously. After proper timeout, cannulas are connected to ECMO circuit and ECMO is initiated. After the achievement of adequate ECMO flows, CPR is stopped. Mild therapeutic hypothermia is achieved for 24–48 hours by cooling the patient to 33–34°C through integrated heat exchanger in the ECMO circuit. Permissive hypothermia reduces the tissue metabolism including cerebral metabolism, giving a better chance of survival of the patient, and reducing the progressive cerebral injury [54–56]. The patient is

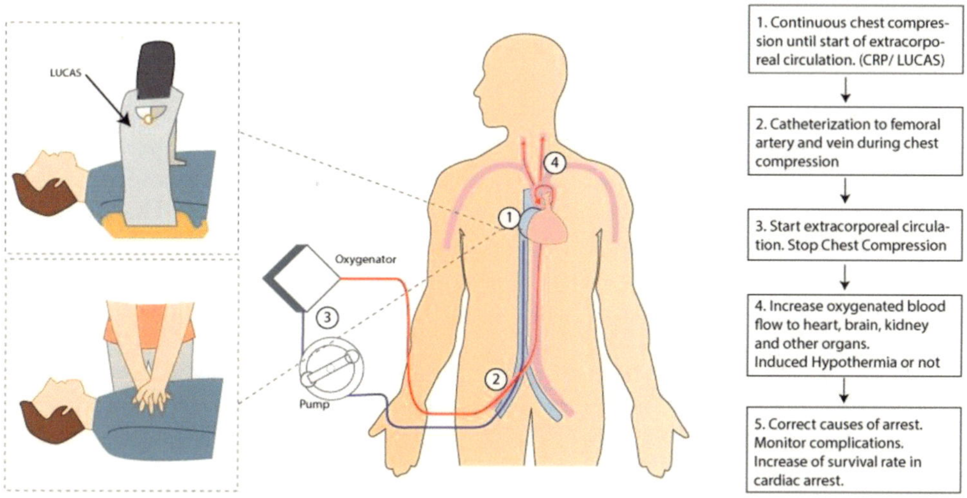

Figure 4.
Steps of institution of ECPR.

connected to the ventilator to reduce the work of breathing. IV heparin is infused for anticoagulation and routine arterial blood gas (ABGs) and lactate monitoring are done to measure the success of ECMO, and mean arterial pressure (MAP) is aimed at 70 mmHg. As soon as a patient is stabilized on ECPR, he should be wheeled to the cath lab for angiography for coronary angiography with or without stenting. To prevent the ischemia in the limb with arterial cannula, 6–7 Fr, arterial cannula is inserted distally and sliced into the arterial cannula allowing perfusion of the distal limb. However, insertion of distal limb perfusion cannula may be extremely challenging in patients with peripheral vascular disease, profound shock with collapsed and constricted arteries, or obesity. The alternative in such patients may be to use retrograde limb perfusion through dorsalis pedis, anterior tibial, or posterior tibial artery. Reports have shown favorable results with retrograde limb perfusion with decreased incidence of leg ischemia and fasciotomy [57, 58]. In patients with small femoral vessels, an alternate technique may be to insert 12 Fr or 14 Fr bilateral femoral arterial cannula instead of a single 17 Fr or 19 Fr arterial cannula. The steps of ECPR are shown in **Figure 4**.

7. Complications of ECPR

ECPR, like other forms of ECLS, is used as a potential lifesaving approach. But it has the potential for adverse consequences ranging from minor to fatal complications. Observational studies show that 1 in 4 patients ends up having complications [59]. Complications include limb ischemia, vascular damage leading to inability to the cannulate the vessel or profound intracorporeal or extracorporeal bleeding, tamponade, failure to maintain adequate ECMO flow resulting in inadequate support, and intracranial hemorrhage with grave consequences and dismal survival. Other issues such as multiple organ failure, sepsis, and hypoxic brain injury (cerebral stroke or cerebral stroke and hemorrhage, coma, diffuse anoxic brain injury, and brain death) can also occur in the absence of adequate perfusion of the organs with oxygenated blood [50, 60].

8. Results

8.1 In-hospital cardiac arrest

Patients who have IHCA are usually witnessed and have high likelihood of a good outcome with CCPR. A considerable proportion of these patients are candidates for ECPR. However, of all patients who had an in-hospital cardiac arrest (IHCA), only less than 1% were treated with ECPR in the United States [61]. With widespread availability and increasing familiarity of physician with ECMO, ECPR is gradually increasing in the past 20 years in a hospital setting. Encouraging results of ECPR for IHCA lead to renewed interest in research in this field with the development of automated CPR tools, percutaneous cannula, and localization of vessels under ultrasound guidance. Even with this limited research, there have been promising results of ECPR on patients who had IHCA with survival rates between 17 and 28% [31, 32]. These survival rates have led to great optimism in ECPR as a treatment for CA. Chen et al. conducted a 3-year prospective observational study using ECLS. The inclusion criteria were patients aged 18–75 years old who had an IHCA of cardiac origin having CPR >10 min compared to patients with CCPR. The prognostic factors in both groups were balanced by propensity score resulting in a comparable cohort, 113 with CCPR, and 59 in the ECPR group. Patients with ECPR had superior 1-year survival and survival to discharge rate, which was also the primary endpoint [62]. Shin et al. from Korea conducted a single-center, retrospective observational study from January 2003 to June 2009. A total of 406 patients had IHCA, broken down into a population getting CCPR (n = 321) vs. ECPR (n = 85). Propensity matching was used to balance the groups, and discharge with minimal neurologic impairment was used as the primary endpoint. ECPR group was superior in the primary endpoint. In addition, survival rates at 6-month survival were statistically significant in ECPR group [63].

8.2 Out-of-hospital cardiac arrest

Encouraging results with IABP in patients with coronary artery disease, cardiogenic shock, and postcardiotomy shock led to use of IABP for resuscitation of patients with CA. However, subsequent studies performed to review the results of IABP in patients with CA failed to show any survival benefit [64]. In a study by Iqbal et al. comparing the effects of IABP in patients with CA (55 patients with IABP vs. 174 without IABP), authors found no difference in favorable functional status at discharge (49.1% in IAPB group vs. 57.1% in without IABP group) and mortality rate at one year (45.5% in IABP group vs. 35.5% in without IABP group) [65]. In a randomized clinical trial by Firduas et al. including 60 patients with CA due to acute coronary syndrome patients (ACS) (30 patients received IABP after CA vs. 30 patients without IABP), there was no difference between the groups in terms of hospital mortality, hospital stay, cell death marker, or improvement in lactate clearance [66].

8.3 Comparison between in-hospital and out-of-hospital cardiac arrest

The length of CA, which is more relevant than the site of CA, is an important variable for the disparity in outcomes. IHCA patients are more likely to witnessed with a shorter time to initiate BLS and ACLS and a shorter period until the initiation of ECMO, as well as that their comorbidities are known to the treating physician, implying a bias in the choice to implant an ECMO. The key element in determining the success of ECPR in a patient with CA is the amount of time elapsed between the occurrence of the CA and initiation of ECMO. In most cases, IHCA would have a shorter time in achieving the ECMO flow as the tools and equipment are more readily available than OHCA. Still, survival to discharge in patients managed with ECPR for OHCA was reported to be significantly higher compared to patients managed with CCPR (56.9% vs. 43.1%, respectively; OR: 1.16, 95% CI: 1.11–1.21, $p < 0.001$) [67, 68]. The CHEER trial (mechanical CPR, Hypothermia, ECMO, and Early Reperfusion), a single center, prospective, observational study done in The Alfred Hospital Australia, included 24 patients with IHCA and OHCA who were eventually put on ECMO. ROSC was seen in all the patients, and more than half could be taken off ECMO, eventually making the survival rate above fifty percent. Neurological recovery was seen in over half of the patients who were discharged from the hospital in similar numbers [54]. Another retrospective review from Canada by Sun et al. in patients who received ECMO for cardiac arrest (8 IHCA, 1 OHCA) or cardiogenic shock (13 patients) from April 2009 to July 2015 at Vancouver General Hospital in Canada reported that ECMO was successfully weaned off in 18 patients and 16 could be discharged. Fifteen patients had satisfactory neurological outcomes [69]. Aforesaid studies demonstrate that in appropriately selected patients, ECPR provides survival benefits and more positive neurological outcomes. In a meta-analysis including 2260 patients from six studies comparing ECPR or CCPR in patients with CA since 2000, Wang et al. reviewed the survival rates and neurological outcomes at discharge and at 3–6 months as well as 1 year after CA. The survival rate to discharge (RR 2.37, 95% CI 1.63–3.45, $P < 0.001$) and good long-term neurological outcome (RR 2.79, 95% CI 1.96–3.97, $P < 0.001$) were significantly better in ECPR group. In subgroup analysis, survival to discharge was significantly better with ECPR over CCPR in OHCA patients (RR 2.69, 95% CI 1.48–4.91, $P = 0.001$), while no significant difference was found in IHCA patients (RR 1.84, 95% CI 0.91–3.73, $P = 0.09$). The patient's survival rate to discharge was 25.5% in patients who received ECPR, and 19.4% of them had good long-term neurological outcomes [70]. Authors concluded that with the availability of facilities using ECPR for IHCA, more patients would survive and have an active life with little neurological deficiency.

8.4 Limitations

ECPR remains a niche procedure that requires trained staff and resources, both of which are only available in tertiary centers with vital ECMO programs. Another problem is deciding which patients should receive ECPR, as the etiology alone is insufficient to foretell survival using ECPR. More multi-institutional studies are necessary to develop better guidelines for ECPR [71]. Presently, ECPR use is mainly limited to the pediatric population as most of the etiology is linked to congenital pathologies and may see better outcomes if ECMO buys enough time for recovery from postcardiotomy myocardial stunning, a transplant, or corrective procedure [72, 73].

9. Conclusion

Over the last several decades, healthcare results for this demographic procedure have improved significantly due to increased expertise and experience in patient care. ECMO remains an invaluable tool in the armamentarium of cardiac surgery, and its use combined with CPR has promising results, but it is hindered by nonavailability and high capital usage from the hospital. ECPR must be judicially used in the context of CA as every case will not lead to successful resuscitation. Surgical and medical management of CA patients continues to be difficult. Despite gains, various learning opportunities remain as we try to make even more progress.

9.1 Role of ECMO in cardiogenic shock due to acute myocardial infarction and nonacute myocardial infarction cardiogenic shock

Acute myocardial infarction (AMI) remains the leading cause of CS. However, non-AMI-related CS is on the rise. Etiologies of cardiogenic shock are enumerated in **Table 3** [74]. The management and response to the intervention vary based on etiology. Despite optimal management, CS continues to be associated with significant morbidity and 30–60% mortality [75]. Various AMCS devices that are available for the management of these patients are IABP, Impella, Protec Duo cannula, CentriMag pump, TandemHeart, and VA-ECMO to provide left- and/or right-heart support [76]. Among all AMCS devices, IABP remains the most widely used, although the use of other more robust devices is increasing [76–78]. Among all the available devices, ECMO provides the highest level of cardiopulmonary support.

Acute myocardial infarction
Mechanical complications related to acute myocardial infarction • Ventricular septal defect • Ischemic mitral regurgitation
Acute on chronic heart failure
Acute right ventricular failure • Right ventricular myocardial infarction • Right ventricular failure after left ventricular assist device
Acute myocarditis
Refractory cardiac arrest
Refractory arrhythmias
Post-cardiotomy shock
Severe valvular heart disease
Post-heart transplant primary graft dysfunction
Stress cardiomyopathy (Takotsubo cardiomyopathy)
Peripartum cardiomyopathy
Cardiac trauma with or without cardiac tamponade
Acute pulmonary embolism
Severe pulmonary hypertension
Drug intoxication
High-risk interventions • Percutaneous coronary intervention • Ventricular tachycardia ablation
Septic shock

Table 3.
Potential indications for acute mechanical circulatory support device in cardiogenic shock.

In the subsequent sections, we will discuss the role of ECMO in CS due to AMI (AMICS) and in the subsequent section, we will discuss the role of ECMO in non-AMI CS including septic shock.

9.2 Role of ECMO in post-acute myocardial infarction cardiogenic shock

Shock is a condition of cellular and tissue hypoxia due to decreased oxygen delivery, increased oxygen demand, or inefficient oxygen utilization, or a combination of these [79]. Acute shock is reversible for a short duration, but it quickly becomes irreversible, leading to multi-organ failure (MOF) and death [80]. Cardiogenic shock (CS) occurs due to cardiac pump failure and defined as a primary cardiac disorder that results in both clinical and biochemical evidences of tissue hypoperfusion including altered mental status, oliguria, and respiratory failure. Clinical criteria include systolic blood pressure (SBP) ≤90 mmHg for ≥30 minutes or need for support to maintain systolic blood pressure ≥90 mmHg and urine output less ≤ 30 mL/h or cool extremities. Hemodynamic criteria include a depressed cardiac index (≤2.2 L/min/m^2

of body surface area) and an elevated pulmonary-capillary wedge pressure (PCWP) >15 mmHg [81, 82].

Acute myocardial infarction complicated by cardiogenic shock (AMICS) is a grievous condition associated with significant morbidity and mortality. In several observational studies in patients with AMI, conservative therapy has >80% mortality [83]. Despite primary percutaneous intervention (PCI) with coronary artery angioplasty has significantly improved the survival and has become standard of care for the management of AMI, no definitive management is available for the patients with AMICS [84]. In patients with AMI, 3–10% patients develop CS. Emergency revascularization does not significantly reduce 30-day mortality but significantly improves the six-month survival and long-term outcome in patients with AMICS [83]. In patients with AMICS, mortality rate is 30–50% with primary PCI and >80% in patients without primary PCI [85–87].

Acute myocardial infarction due to acute myocardial ischemia results in severe systolic and diastolic dysfunction of the heart with elevation in left ventricular end-diastolic pressure (LVEDP), PCWP, pulmonary edema, decrease in stroke volume, and low cardiac output [88]. Therefore, the aim of treating AMICS patients is to alleviate myocardial ischemia, reduce ventricular loading, support cardiac and respiratory function, and improve end-organ perfusion [89].

Given the high early mortality rate associated with AMICS despite revascularization therapies, physicians have sought out other therapies to improve results. Advancement in the technology has expanded the availability of acute mechanical circulatory support (AMCS) devices such as intra-aortic balloon pump (IABP), Impella, and ECMO. IABP was the earliest available AMCS device. Positive impact in improving coronary and systemic perfusion and reducing the myocardial oxygen demand in the setting of heart failure reported in various animal and human studies in the late 1990s and early 2000s led to widespread use of IABP in patients with AMI [90, 91]. The SHOCK (Should We Emergently Revascularize Occluded Coronaries for Cardiogenic Shock) registry also showed >15% reduction in in-hospital mortality with use of IABP in patients with AMI who underwent thrombolysis (46.5% in thrombolysis and IABP vs. 62.9% in thrombolysis alone, $P < 0.005$). However, when the SHOCK Trial and Registry established the significant impact of early revascularization with percutaneous coronary intervention (PCI) or coronary artery bypass grafting (CABG) on the survival in patients with AMI, use of IABP went into disrepute [83, 92]. Subsequent IABP-SHOCK II (Intra-aortic Balloon Support for Myocardial Infarction with Cardiogenic Shock) trial in 2012 that included 600 patients failed to demonstrate any benefit of IABP over medical therapy alone immediately prior to coronary revascularization in terms of reduced 30-day mortality, achieving hemodynamic stability, ICU stay, organ perfusion, dose of catecholamine, rate of stroke, bleeding, peripheral ischemic complications, recurrent AMI, and stent thrombosis [93]. Further 12-month and 6-year follow-ups of SHOCK-IABP II trial patients also did not show any mortality benefit [94, 95]. All of these led to downgradation of IABP use in patients with AMI-CS to class IIIB in the European Society of Cardiology and class IIb recommendation in the American College of Cardiology/American Heart Association guidelines [96, 97]. Subsequently, use of other AMCS devices has increased for the management of AMICS. In last decade, Impella has become the most commonly used device after IABP in patients with AMICS with LV dysfunction for periprocedural management. However, in patients with biventricular failure, associated respiratory distress or acute respiratory distress syndrome (ARDS), and mechanical complications of AMI such as mitral regurgitation or ventricular septal defect, ECMO is preferred over other devices. In resource-limited countries where other AMCS devices are not available apart from IABP and ECMO, ECMO can be used for periprocedural management. Further, ECMO is the only AMCS device that provides complete cardiopulmonary support and improves end-organ perfusion. Studies have also supported the role of ECMO in the management of AMICS patients. A study by Sheu et al. including patients with AMICS who underwent primary PCI without the ECMO (115 patients) and primary PCI with ECMO (219 patients) found significantly reduced 30-day mortality (30.1% for ECMO group vs. 41.7% for non-ECMO group) with the use of ECMO [98]. Another study by Tsao et al. also evaluated the role of ECMO in patients with AMICS and managed with primary PCI. The first group managed with IABP (25 patients), and the second group managed with ECMO (33 patients). Baseline characteristics and disease severity including age, gender, coronary risk factors, TIMI risk scores for STEMI and NSTEMI, euro SCORE, APACHE score, and SYNTAX score (including the number of coronary vessels that were involved) were comparable in both the groups. Patients in the ECMO group had significantly increased survival compared to IABP group (44% in IABP group vs. 81.82% in ECMO group), and this trend continued through the 1-year follow-up (survival in IABP group 24% vs. survival in ECMO group 63.64%) [99]. A retrospective single-center study done by Esper et al. included 18 patients who received VA-ECMO for AMICS, after the revascularization therapy. ECMO run lasted for an average of 3.2 ± 2.5 days with a mean hospital stay of 23.4 days, and 67% of patients survived to discharge [100].

Another study by Negi et al. included 15 patients with AMI and refractory CS who were placed on VA-ECMO. One-third of these patients had OHCA and 60% had ST elevated AMI. In 60% of patients, IABP was inserted in addition to VA-ECMO. Median duration of VA-ECMO support was 45 hours, and 50% of patients were successfully weaned off VA-ECMO. The survival to discharge was 47%, and all survivors were alive 30 days after discharge. In total, 53% of patients experienced vascular complications [101]. Another observational study by Vallabhajosyula et al. utilizing the National Inpatient Sample database also reported 40.8% survival with use of VA-ECMO in patients with AMICS. The study analyzed 2962 patients over a period of 14 years. There was a notable trend toward improving survival over the course of time, and 12% of patients were bridged to a left ventricular assist device (LVAD) or heart transplantation [102]. A systematic review of nine studies of patients with acute myocardial infection-induced cardiac shock concluded that using venoarterial extracorporeal membrane oxygenation provides temporary support has more benefits compared to standards of care and can assure a higher survival rate [103].

Although various retrospective observational studies support the role of ECMO in the management of patients with AMICS, there have been no randomized controlled trials (RCTs) assessing the use of ECMO in AMICS. Currently, two European RCTs, EURO-SHOCK, and ECLS-SHOCK, are enrolling the patients. EURO-SHOCK will randomly assign 428 patients to ECMO or conventional therapy and evaluate 30-day mortality as the primary result; the study is anticipated to conclude in February 2024 [104]. ECLS SHOCK will also randomize 420 patients with AMICS undergoing revascularization to ECMO or medical treatment alone. The primary outcome is 30-day mortality, and the trial is anticipated to conclude in August 2023 [105].

9.3 Role of ECMO in nonacute myocardial infarction cardiogenic shock

Patients with acute heart failure (HF) who present in CS have high mortality. Conventional HF therapies including optimal medical management, inotropes, vasopressors, and IABP are the initial line of management. However, patients who fail to respond to medical management may benefit from VA-ECMO. It is indicated in patients with medically refractory CS and in patients at high risk of cardiogenic shock as determined by scoring systems such as CardShock risk score and IABP-SHOCK II risk scores. ECMO is also AMCS of choice in patients with CS who have biventricular failure, respiratory failure, life-threatening arrhythmias, or cardiac arrest. There is often an overlap between indications for ECMO and AMCS devices. However, patients with CS who have associated respiratory failure are best managed by ECMO [106, 107]. The outcome of ECMO in patients with HF varies significantly depending on the etiology. The survival after hospital discharge for patients managed with ECMO is 71.9% for myocarditis [108], 74.3% for patients with primary graft failure post-heart transplant [109], and 42% one-year survival for patients with acute decompensation of chronic cardiomyopathy. However, patients aged >75 years, patients with severe neurological injury, multiple organ failure, and multiple comorbidities are risk factors for adverse outcomes. Dangers et al. also reported poor outcomes of ECMO in patients with SOFA scores >13 prior to ECMO cannulation [110].

The role of ECMO in these patients varies depending upon the etiology and can be a bridge to recovery, bridge to transplant, bridge to left ventricular assist device (VAD), or bridge to decision [111].

1. Bridge to recovery (BTR): ECMO weaning rates are reported as 75.5% in patients with acute myocarditis, 87% for patients with primary graft failure after heart transplant, and 55% for AMICS. In most cases, recovery occurs within a week, and if recovery does not occur, the strategy must be changed to bridge to bridge (BTB) or Bridge to transplant (BTT) [108, 109, 112].

2. Bridge to bridge (BTB): Patients with CS due to acute on chronic heart failure are often bridged to durable VAD (the durable VAD itself may serve as bridge to transplantation). It is important to make the decision early to bridge to VAD after patient stabilizes on ECMO if there is no recovery of cardiac function [113, 114].

3. Bridge to transplant (BTT): With the availability of other robust percutaneous AMCS devices, it has become rare to use ECMO as a bridge to transplant, especially in adult patients as other AMCS devices are easier to manage and can be kept for longer duration without significant complications compared to ECMO.

4. Bridge to decision: Patients having acute decompensation with CS, especially with unknown neurological status, can be acutely managed with ECMO. This provides sufficient time for evaluation, intervention, and decision for further management while the heart and rest of the body are supported with ECMO. The decision of further management can be taken based on the recovery of organ function and neurological status.

9.4 Advantages of ECMO in cardiogenic shock

1. Easy and rapid insertion: Time is an essence for a patient rapidly deteriorating due to CS. ECMO can be placed rapidly percutaneously with Seldinger technique using ultrasound at the patient's bedside, in the cath lab, in the operating room, and in the field. Even nonsurgeon medical personnel can insert an ECMO in the prehospital setting without compromising safety [115].

2. Provides complete cardiac support: With flow rates of up to 6 L/min, ECMO can completely replace native heart function in patients with profound CS [116].

3. Biventricular support: Almost 38–45% patients with AMICS develop acute RV failure and patients with chronic cardiomyopathy, post-cardiotomy also develop acute heart failure. Among all the available AMCS devices, only ECMO can provide complete biventricular support [117].

4. Respiratory support: In patients with ARDS with secondary Takotsubo syndrome and patients with CS having associated respiratory failure, increased pulmonary airway pressure can adversely affect the failing right heart. ECMO by providing complete cardiorespiratory support provide an opportunity to keep the ventilator at rest setting allowing the lungs to recover without barotrauma and preventing the adverse effect of high positive end-expiratory pressure on the right ventricle.

5. Effective in life-threatening arrhythmias*:* Uncontrollable arrhythmias, such as incessant ventricular tachycardia (VT storm), can be managed with ECMO by reducing myocardial stroke work and improving coronary perfusion, and patient can undergo ablation of VT focus in the cath lab on ECMO support [81].

6. Cardiogenic shock complicated by refractory cardiac arrest: CardShock study showed that 28% of patients with CS suffer from cardiac arrest. The use of ECMO in patients with witnessed refractory CA has been shown to improve survival [118].

7. Portable: Miniaturized ECMO machine is easy to transport on the ground as well as air ambulance.

9.5 Disadvantages of ECMO in cardiogenic shock

1. Left ventricular (LV) distension: ECMO drains the blood from the right atrial, but, has no direct effect on the left side of the heart. Due to the absence of reservoir, smaller size of venous cannula, significantly amount of blood escapes the venous drainage and reaches the left heart. Further, blood returning to the left atrium vis. Thebesian veins, bronchial veins draining into the pulmonary veins, and blood returning to the LV due to aortic regurgitation also reach the left ventricle. Further, ECMO increases LV afterload by retrogradely flowing the blood into the ascending aorta. The heart with severely reduced contractility is unable to overcome this afterload, and the aortic valve remains closed. These patients are at risk of left ventricular distention, left atrial hypertension, and pulmonary edema [119].

2. Complications: Due to the large size of arterial and venous cannula, patients are at risk of vascular injury and injury to the heart. A meta-analysis reported 40.8% incidence of bleeding, 30.4% incidence of infection, 5.8% incidence of stroke, and 4.7% incidence of lower limb amputation [60]. The cannulation site is the most common site for bleeding [109, 120]. In a Japanese study, use of smaller cannula in small caliber vessels was associated with reduced risk of bleeding without compromising the outcome [121]. A meta-analysis of 22 cohort studies also found that distal perfusion cannulas reduced the limb ischemia by 15.7% [122]. Another devastating complication of ECMO is intracranial hemorrhage as patients on VA-ECMO are anticoagulated with heparin or bivalirudin. In a large study of adult patients with intracranial bleeds after ECMO, low platelets were independently associated with an increased risk of bleeding [123]. The risk of inter-cranial bleeding increased significantly at platelet counts below 50,000/cc. Therefore, it is recommended to maintain the platelet counts ≥100,000/cc while a patient is on ECMO [124].

The outcome of ECMO can be improved by using smaller cannula in small vessels, more liberal use of LV venting, routine use of distal limp perfusion cannula, and maintaining adequate platelet counts. SAVE and ENCOURAGE score systems, which are used in pre-ECMO patient variables to predict outcomes, may help in better patient selection for this risky but life-saving intervention [125].

9.6 Sepsis-induced cardiomyopathy and Use of ECMO

Sepsis is a potentially life-threatening condition that occurs due to systemic dysregulated inflammation secondary to overwhelming infection, which affects various organs [125]. An important complication of severe sepsis is sepsis-induced cardiomyopathy (SIC), which is reversible depression of myocardium [126]. This occurs due to structural damage and dysfunction of the myocardium caused by widespread inflammatory cytokine release and mitochondrial dysfunction [127]. There are three characteristics of SIC: dilation of the left ventricle (LV), reduced EF (ejection fraction), and reversibility of cardiomyopathy in 7–10 days after the resolution of sepsis [128]. With improvement in the understanding of molecular biology, our understanding of SIC has significantly improved in last few decades. Although the use of ECMO is increasing in the treatment of various cardiac and noncardiac conditions, it has not been treated as standard practice protocol for adult patients with septic shock, unlike pediatric and neonatal patients [129–132]. Despite the ECMO has gained wide acceptance for the treatment of adult respiratory distress syndrome (ARDS), the effectiveness of ECMO in treating septic shock still remains controversial [129, 133]. In this section, we will discuss SIC and the viability of ECMO as a treatment option.

9.7 Mechanism of sepsis-induced cardiomyopathy

There are two different mechanisms proposed for the etiopathogenesis of SIC. First, based on animal studies, insufficient coronary blood flow is supposed to cause myocardial ischemia [134]. Second, due to the surge of chemical mediators such as cytokines, endotoxins, and nitric oxide (NO) that are released during the dysregulated inflammation may cause SIC. However, in a study done by Cunnion et al, measuring coronary blood flow and myocardial metabolism using coronary sinus thermodilution catheters in seven patients with septic shock to determine whether myocardial depression was associated with reduced coronary flow [135]; the authors found that coronary blood flow was similar or higher in the patients with septic shock compared to the controls despite the presence of myocardial depression. A recent study by Rudiger and Singer has also shown that SIC cannot be attributed to the disruption in coronary circulation [128].

The role of chemical mediators has also been studied extensively in the pathophysiology of SIC. Studies have implicated the role of endotoxins, interleukin-1β (IL-1β), and tumor necrosis factor-alpha (TNF-α) in the pathogenesis of SIC [136–138]. Endotoxins induce NO synthase and increase the production and release of NO [136]. Similarly, cytokines such as TNF-α and IL-1β also increase the activity of cyclic guanosine monophosphate (cGMP) and NO [138]. It has been hypothesized that excess NO production causes cardiac dysfunction by reducing the myofibril response to calcium, dysfunction of the mitochondria, and downregulation of β-adrenergic receptors [128, 139, 140]. Several studies have also suggested that NO overproduction and mitochondrial dysfunction may contribute to cardiac dysfunction and mortality [141–144]. Interestingly, using methylene blue an inhibitor of NO production pathway has demonstrated improvement in myocardial depression, maintenance of oxygen transportation, and reduction in the requirement for concurrent adrenergic support [145].

9.8 Diagnosis, treatment options and use of ECMO

There is a range of tests that are available for diagnosing SIC. These include blood tests such as brain natriuretic peptide (BNP) assay and Troponin Assay as well as use of echocardiogram to check for ventricular dysfunction. While BNP and troponin I, both rise in SIC, their rise is mainly dependent on the severity of illness rather than markers for cardiomyopathy [146–148]. The gold standard for the diagnosis of SIC is echocardiography. Echocardiogram may show normal or reduced ejection fraction, LV diastolic dysfunction, and RV systolic dysfunction, as well as global longitudinal strain (GLS) on myocardial speckle tracking [149–152].

9.9 Improved outcome of patients with sepsis-induced cardiomyopathy and use of ECMO

While the management of SIC has been previously limited to vasopressors, inotropes, and fluid management, the use of ECMO has recently been explored. A low cardiac output due to SIC can impair the organ perfusion and precipitate multi-organ failure. Thus, it appears reasonable to identify and restore the cardiac output in these patients. Patients deteriorating despite maximal pharmacological support should be promptly transitioned to acute mechanical circulatory support (AMCS) device including VA-ECMO. Studies have found that VA-ECMO significantly improves the survival in patients with SIC with LV dysfunction compared to patients with preserved LV function [153, 154].

An important multicenter retrospective study performed by Bréchot et al. and published in 2020 investigated the role of VA-ECMO in patients with SIC. In this study, 82 patients with a sepsis-induced refractory shock treated with VA-ECMO were compared to 130 patients treated with conventional therapy for 90 days. Despite a propensity-weighted analysis, survival in the treatment group was higher than that in the control group (51% vs. 14%, relative risk for mortality 0.57, $p = 0.003$). The study also concluded that survival with VA-ECMO was better in younger patients and the strong initial protective effect of VA-ECMO waned over time [(0 to 7 days: HR 0.14; 95% CI: 0.05 to 0.41) vs. (7 to 14 days: HR 0.79; 95% CI: 0.13 to 4.64)] [155]. The findings of the study emphasized that patients with SIC should be identified and supported with VA-ECMO as early as possible.

9.10 Patient selection for ECMO

In patients with sepsis, 13–65% develop SCM, but not all patients in septic shock will benefit from VA-ECMO [153, 156–158]. Patients with sepsis who are refractory to standard therapy, including adequate fluid resuscitation, antibiotics, and stress dose steroids, have increasing requirement of vasopressors and inotropes, and echocardiography findings are consistent with SCM, and they should be considered for prompt VA-ECMO support. A positive blood culture alone is not a contraindication for VA-ECMO, especially when source control and antibiotic therapy have already been initiated [159]. The early introduction of VA-ECMO and other types of MCS can prevent adverse effects of an escalating dose of inotropes and vasopressors and the mechanical ventilation, the effect termed as “metabolic rest” [160]. Any situation in which incremental escalation of standard therapies results in disproportionately lower hemodynamic improvement should warrant the use of ECMO and other AMCS devices. However, use of ECMO in patients with SCM who had CA remains controversial with poor outcomes [161, 162].

9.11 Concurrent management along with ECMO

In a patient with SCM supported by VA-ECMO, apart from managing ECMO, other important goals are augmentation of cardiac output, ventilator management, anticoagulation, and hemodynamic support [163]. Ventilation parameters should promote “lung rest” by offloading the mechanical power required for oxygenation and ventilation by the lungs [164]. Peak inspiratory pressure should be maintained <25 cmH2O and minimizes FiO2 while maintaining 5–12 cmH2O of positive end expiratory pressure (PEEP) to prevent atelectasis [165]. For anticoagulation, heparin is most commonly used and recommended by ELSO [166]; however, use of bivalirudin has been found to be associated with reduced mortality in adult patients [167]. For hemodynamic management, these patients are usually vasoplegic due to both septic shock and VA-ECMO and need vasopressors such as norepinephrine, phenylephrine,

Pros	Cons
1. Fully restores cardiac output [167]. 2. Decompresses right ventricle [170]. 3. Provide adequate pulmonary support [164].	1. Resource and personnel intensive to manage ECMO. 2. Risk of LV distension due to increased systemic afterload especially in peripheral configuration [19]. 3. Risk of ischemia of lower extremity (distal perfusion cannulation may alleviate this) [171]. 4. The risk of cerebral hypoxemia (North-South Syndrome) [172]. 5. Risk of heparin-induced thrombo-cytopenia (HIT) in patients receiving heparin as anticoagulant [173].

Table 4.
Pros and cons of using VA-ECMO in patients with septic cardiomyopathy.

vasopressin, and epinephrine to counteract vasoplegia. In case of suboptimal effect, agents such as methylene blue, hydroxycobalamin, and angiotensin II should be considered [168, 169].

Pros and Cons of VA-ECMO in sepsis-induced cardiomyopathy: While it has been established that ECMO is a viable option for management of SCM, **Table 4** presents the pros and cons of ECMO in patients with septic cardiomyopathy.

Author details

Pankaj Garg[1], John H. Yazji[2], Emad Alamouti-Fard[2], Ishaq Wadiwala[2], Mohammad Alomari[2], Md Walid Akram Hussain[2], Mohamed Samir Hassan Elawady[2], Saqib Masroor[3] and Samuel Jacob[4]*

1 Cardiothoracic Surgery, Mayo Clinic, Jacksonville, Florida, USA

2 Cardiothoracic Surgery Research Unit, Mayo Clinic, Jacksonville, Florida, USA

3 Cardiothoracic Surgery, University of Toledo, Ohio, USA

4 Clinical Research Director Heart and Lung Transplant Program, Mayo Clinic, Florida, USA

*Address all correspondence to: jacob.samuel@mayo.edu

References

[1] MacLaren G, Combes A, Bartlett RH. Contemporary extracorporeal membrane oxygenation for adult respiratory failure: Life support in the new era. Intensive Care Medicine. 2012;**38**(2):210-220

[2] Kluge S, Braune SA, Engel M, Nierhaus A, Frings D, Ebelt H, et al. Avoiding invasive mechanical ventilation by extracorporeal carbon dioxide removal in patients failing noninvasive ventilation. Intensive Care Medicine. 2012;**38**(10):1632-1639

[3] Frenckner B. Extracorporeal membrane oxygenation: A breakthrough for respiratory failure. Journal of Internal Medicine. 2015;**278**(6):586-598

[4] Kolff WJ, Berk HT, ter Welle M, van der Ley AJ, van Dijk EC, van Noordwijk J. The artificial kidney: A dialyser with a great area. Journal of the American Society of Nephrology. 1997;**8**(12):1959-1965

[5] Gibbon JH Jr. Application of a mechanical heart and lung apparatus to cardiac surgery. Minnesota Medicine. 1954;**37**(3):171-185

[6] Cohn LH. Fifty years of open-heart surgery. Circulation. 2003;**107**(17):2168-2170

[7] Kirklin JW, Dushane JW, Patrick RT, Donald DE, Hetzel PS, Harshbarger HG, et al. Intracardiac surgery with the aid of a mechanical pump-oxygenator system (gibbon type): Report of eight cases. Proceedings of the Staff Meetings. Mayo Clinic. 1955;**30**(10):201-206

[8] Hill JD, O'Brien TG, Murray JJ, Dontigny L, Bramson ML, Osborn JJ, et al. Prolonged extracorporeal oxygenation for acute post-traumatic respiratory failure (shock-lung syndrome). Use of the Bramson membrane lung. The New England Journal of Medicine. 1972;**286**(12):629-634

[9] Bartlett RH, Gazzaniga AB, Fong SW, Burns NE. Prolonged extracorporeal cardiopulmonary support in man. The Journal of Thoracic and Cardiovascular Surgery. 1974;**68**(6):918-932

[10] Hicks RE, Kinney TR, Raphaely RC, Donaldson MH, Edmunds LH Jr, Naiman JL. Successful treatment of varicella pneumonia with prolonged extracorporeal membrane oxygenation in a child with leukemia. The Journal of Thoracic and Cardiovascular Surgery. 1977;**73**(2):297-302

[11] Chauhan S, Subin S. Extracorporeal membrane oxygenation, an anesthesiologist's perspective: Physiology and principles. Part 1. Annals of Cardiac Anaesthesia. 2011;**14**(3):218-229

[12] Reichman RT, Joyo CI, Dembitsky WP, Griffith LD, Adamson RM, Daily PO, et al. Improved patient survival after cardiac arrest using a cardiopulmonary support system. The Annals of Thoracic Surgery. 1990;**49**(1):101-104

[13] Ruszel N, Kiełbowski K, Piotrowska M, Kubisa M, Grodzki T, Wójcik J, et al. Central, peripheral ECMO or CPB? Comparison between circulatory support methods used during lung transplantation. Journal of Cardiothoracic Surgery. 2021;**16**(1):341

[14] Pavlushkov E, Berman M, Valchanov K. Cannulation techniques for extracorporeal life support. Annals of Translational Medicine. 2017;**5**(4):70

[15] Tsangaris A, Alexy T, Kalra R, Kosmopoulos M, Elliott A,

Bartos JA, et al. Overview of veno-arterial extracorporeal membrane oxygenation (VA-ECMO) support for the management of cardiogenic shock. Frontiers in Cardiovascular Medicine. 2021;**8**:686558

[16] Fuhrman BP, Hernan LJ, Rotta AT, Heard CM, Rosenkranz ER. Pathophysiology of cardiac extracorporeal membrane oxygenation. Artificial Organs. 1999;**23**:966-969

[17] Kalra R, Kosmopoulos M, Goslar T, Raveendran G, Bartos JA, Yannopoulos D. Extracorporeal cardiopulmonary resuscitation for cardiac arrest. Current Opinion in Critical Care. 2020;**26**:228-235

[18] Kosmopoulos M, Kalra R, Bartos JA, Raveendran G, Yannopoulos D. Contemporary approaches to cardiopulmonary resuscitation: Physiology-guided approaches. Journal of Emergency and Critical Care Medicine. 2019;**4**:19

[19] Cevasco M, Takayama H, Ando M, Garan AR, Naka Y, Takeda K. Left ventricular distension and venting strategies for patients on venoarterial extracorporeal membrane oxygenation. Journal of Thoracic Disease. 2019;**11**(4):1676-1683

[20] Rajagopal K. Left ventricular distension in veno-arterial extracorporeal membrane oxygenation: From mechanics to therapies. ASAIO Journal. 2019;**65**:1-10

[21] Truby LK, Takeda K, Mauro C, Yuzefpolskaya M, Garan AR, Kirtane AJ, et al. Incidence and implications of left ventricular distention during venoarterial extracorporeal membrane oxygenation support. ASAIO Journal. 2017;**63**(3):257-265

[22] Akanni OJ, Takeda K, Truby LK, Kurlansky PA, Chiuzan C, Han J, et al. EC-VAD: Combined use of extracorporeal membrane oxygenation and percutaneous microaxial pump left ventricular assist device. ASAIO Journal. 2019;**65**(3):219-226

[23] Takeda K, Garan AR, Ando M, Han J, Topkara VK, Kurlansky P, et al. Minimally invasive CentriMag ventricular assist device support integrated with extracorporeal membrane oxygenation in cardiogenic shock patients: A comparison with conventional CentriMag biventricular support configuration. European Journal of Cardio-Thoracic Surgery. 2017;**52**(6):1055-1061

[24] Patel SM, Lipinski J, Al-Kindi SG, Patel T, Saric P, Li J, et al. Simultaneous venoarterial extracorporeal membrane oxygenation and percutaneous left ventricular decompression therapy with Impella is associated with improved outcomes in refractory cardiogenic shock. ASAIO Journal. 2019;**65**(1):21-28

[25] Tepper S, Masood MF, Baltazar Garcia M, Pisani M, Ewald GA, Lasala JM, et al. Left ventricular unloading by impella device versus surgical vent during extracorporeal life support. The Annals of Thoracic Surgery. 2017;**104**(3):861-867

[26] Pappalardo F, Schulte C, Pieri M, Schrage B, Contri R, Soeffker G, et al. Concomitant implantation of Impella® on top of veno-arterial extracorporeal membrane oxygenation may improve survival of patients with cardiogenic shock. European Journal of Heart Failure. 2017;**19**(3):404-412

[27] Klee TE, Kern KB. A review of ECMO for cardiac arrest. Resusc Plus. 2021;**5**:100083

[28] Blewer AL, Buckler DG, Li J, Leary M, Becker LB, Shea JA, et al.

Impact of the 2010 resuscitation guidelines training on layperson chest compressions. World Journal of Emergency Medicine. 2015;**6**(4):270-276

[29] Meaney PA, Bobrow BJ, Mancini ME, Christenson J, de Caen AR, Bhanji F, et al. Cardiopulmonary resuscitation quality: [corrected] improving cardiac resuscitation outcomes both inside and outside the hospital: A consensus statement from the American Heart Association. Circulation. 2013;**128**(4):417-435

[30] Yan S, Gan Y, Jiang N, Wang R, Chen Y, Luo Z, et al. The global survival rate among adult out-of-hospital cardiac arrest patients who received cardiopulmonary resuscitation: A systematic review and meta-analysis. Critical Care. 2020;**24**(1):61

[31] Peberdy MA, Kaye W, Ornato JP, Larkin GL, Nadkarni V, Mancini ME, et al. Cardiopulmonary resuscitation of adults in the hospital: A report of 14720 cardiac arrests from the National Registry of Cardiopulmonary Resuscitation. Resuscitation. 2003;**58**(3):297-308

[32] Tonna JE, Selzman CH, Girotra S, Presson AP, Thiagarajan RR, Becker LB, et al. Resuscitation using ECPR during In-hospital cardiac arrest (RESCUE-IHCA) mortality prediction score and external validation. JACC. Cardiovascular Interventions. 2022;**15**(3):237-247

[33] Panchal AR, Berg KM, Hirsch KG, Kudenchuk PJ, Del Rios M, Cabañas JG, et al. 2019 American Heart Association focused update on advanced cardiovascular life support: Use of advanced airways, vasopressors, and extracorporeal cardiopulmonary resuscitation during cardiac arrest: An update to the American Heart Association guidelines for cardiopulmonary resuscitation and emergency cardiovascular care. Circulation. 2019;**140**(24):e881-e894

[34] Swol J, Belohlávek J, Haft JW, Ichiba S, Lorusso R, Peek GJ. Conditions and procedures for in-hospital extracorporeal life support (ECLS) in cardiopulmonary resuscitation (CPR) of adult patients. Perfusion. 2016;**31**(3):182-188

[35] D'Arrigo S, Cacciola S, Dennis M, Jung C, Kagawa E, Antonelli M, et al. Predictors of favourable outcome after in-hospital cardiac arrest treated with extracorporeal cardiopulmonary resuscitation: A systematic review and meta-analysis. Resuscitation. 2017;**121**:62-70

[36] Ryu JA, Cho YH, Sung K, Choi SH, Yang JH, Choi JH, et al. Predictors of neurological outcomes after successful extracorporeal cardiopulmonary resuscitation. BMC Anesthesiology. 2015;**15**:26

[37] Maekawa K, Tanno K, Hase M, Mori K, Asai Y. Extracorporeal cardiopulmonary resuscitation for patients with out-of-hospital cardiac arrest of cardiac origin: A propensity-matched study and predictor analysis. Critical Care Medicine. 2013;**41**(5):1186-1196

[38] Delhomme C, Njeim M, Varlet E, Pechmajou L, Benameur N, Cassan P, et al. Automated external defibrillator use in out-of-hospital cardiac arrest: Current limitations and solutions. Archives of Cardiovascular Diseases. 2019;**112**(3):217-222

[39] Thiagarajan RR, Laussen PC, Rycus PT, Bartlett RH, Bratton SL. Extracorporeal membrane oxygenation to aid cardiopulmonary resuscitation in infants and children. Circulation. 2007;**116**(15):1693-1700

[40] Thiagarajan RR, Brogan TV, Scheurer MA, Laussen PC, Rycus PT, Bratton SL. Extracorporeal membrane oxygenation to support cardiopulmonary resuscitation in adults. The Annals of Thoracic Surgery. 2009;**87**(3):778-785

[41] De Charrière A, Assouline B, Scheen M, et al. ECMO in cardiac arrest: A narrative review of the literature. Journal of Clinical Medicine. 2021;**10**(3):534

[42] Jaski BE, Ortiz B, Alla KR, Smith SC Jr, Glaser D, Walsh C, et al. A 20-year experience with urgent percutaneous cardiopulmonary bypass for salvage of potential survivors of refractory cardiovascular collapse. The Journal of Thoracic and Cardiovascular Surgery. 2010;**139**(3):753

[43] Bartos JA, Yannopoulos D. Refractory cardiac arrest: Where extracorporeal cardiopulmonary resuscitation fits. Current Opinion in Critical Care. 2020;**26**(6):596-602

[44] Bellezzo JM, Shinar Z, Davis DP, Jaski BE, Chillcott S, Stahovich M, et al. Emergency physician-initiated extracorporeal cardiopulmonary resuscitation. Resuscitation. 2012;**83**(8):966-970

[45] Bellezzo J, Shinar Z, Weingart S. Indications and Contraindications of ECLS. EDECMO. Crashing Patient LLC. Retrieved 26 April 2015

[46] Kim H, Cho YH. Role of extracorporeal cardiopulmonary resuscitation in adults. Acute Critical Care. 2020;**35**(1):1-9

[47] Ismail A, Semien G, Miskolczi SY. Cardiopulmonary Bypass. StatPearls: StatPearls Publishing; 2021

[48] Hessel EA 2nd. A brief history of cardiopulmonary bypass. Seminars in Cardiothoracic and Vascular Anesthesia. 2014;**18**(2):87-100

[49] Jastremski MS, Matthias HD, Randell PA. Femoral venous catheterization during cardiopulmonary resuscitation: A critical appraisal. The Journal of Emergency Medicine. 1984;**1**(5):387-391

[50] Conrad SA. Extracorporeal cardiopulmonary resuscitation. The Egyptian Journal of Critical Care Medicine. 2016;**4**(1):11-15

[51] Kumar KM. ECPR-extracorporeal cardiopulmonary resuscitation. Indian Journal of Thoracic Cardiovascular Surgery. 2021;**37**(Suppl. 2):294-302

[52] Akıncı D, Ergun O, Topel Ç, et al. Pelvic abscess drainage: Outcome with factors affecting the clinical success. Diagnostic and Interventional Radiology. 2018;**24**(3):146-152

[53] Banfi C, Pozzi M, Brunner ME, et al. Veno-arterial extracorporeal membrane oxygenation: An overview of different cannulation techniques. Journal of Thoracic Disease. 2016;**8**(9):E875-E885

[54] Stub D, Bernard S, Pellegrino V, Smith K, Walker T, Sheldrake J, et al. Refractory cardiac arrest treated with mechanical CPR, hypothermia, ECMO and early reperfusion (the CHEER trial). Resuscitation. 2015;**86**:88-94

[55] Bernard SA, Gray TW, Buist MD, Jones BM, Silvester W, Gutteridge G, et al. Treatment of comatose survivors of out-of-hospital cardiac arrest with induced hypothermia. The New England Journal of Medicine. 2002;**346**(8):557-563

[56] Hypothermia after Cardiac Arrest Study Group. Mild therapeutic hypothermia to improve the neurologic outcome after cardiac arrest. The

New England Journal of Medicine. 2002;**346**(8):549-556

[57] Göbölös L, Hogan M, Kakar V, Raposo N, Sänger S, Bhatnagar G, et al. Alternative option for limb reperfusion cannula placement for percutaneous femoral veno-arterial ECMO. Perfusion. 2021;**2021**:2676

[58] Rastan AJ, Dege A, Mohr M, Doll N, Falk V, Walther T, et al. Early and late outcomes of 517 consecutive adult patients treated with extracorporeal membrane oxygenation for refractory postcardiotomy cardiogenic shock. The Journal of Thoracic and Cardiovascular Surgery. 2010;**139**(2):302

[59] Jones D, Hilton A, Bellomo R. Extracorporeal membrane oxygenation for inhospital cardiac arrests: The rise of the machines. Critical Care and Resuscitation. 2015;**17**(1):3-5

[60] Cheng R, Hachamovitch R, Kittleson M, Patel J, Arabia F, Moriguchi J, et al. Complications of extracorporeal membrane oxygenation for treatment of cardiogenic shock and cardiac arrest: A meta-analysis of 1,866 adult patients. The Annals of Thoracic Surgery. 2014;**97**(2):610-616

[61] Tonna JE, Selzman CH, Girotra S, Presson AP, Thiagarajan RR, Becker LB, et al. Patient and institutional characteristics influence the decision to use extracorporeal cardiopulmonary resuscitation for in-hospital cardiac arrest. Journal of the American Heart Association. 2020;**9**(9):e01522

[62] Chen YS, Lin JW, Yu HY, Ko WJ, Jerng JS, Chang WT, et al. Cardiopulmonary resuscitation with assisted extracorporeal life-support versus conventional cardiopulmonary resuscitation in adults with in-hospital cardiac arrest: An observational study and propensity analysis. Lancet. 2008;**372**(9638):554-561

[63] Shin TG, Choi JH, Jo IJ, Sim MS, Song HG, Jeong YK, et al. Extracorporeal cardiopulmonary resuscitation in patients with in hospital cardiac arrest: A comparison with conventional cardiopulmonary resuscitation. Critical Care Medicine. 2011;**39**(1):1-7

[64] Mosier JM, Kelsey M, Raz Y, Gunnerson KJ, Meyer R, Hypes CD, et al. Extracorporeal membrane oxygenation (ECMO) for critically ill adults in the emergency department: History, current applications, and future directions. Critical Care. 2015;**19**:431

[65] Iqbal MB, Al-Hussaini A, Rosser G, Rajakulasingam R, Patel J, Elliott K, et al. Intra-aortic balloon pump counterpulsation in the post-resuscitation period is associated with improved functional outcomes in patients surviving an out-of-hospital cardiac arrest: Insights from a dedicated heart attack centre. Heart, Lung & Circulation. 2016;**25**(12):1210-1217

[66] Firdaus I, Yuniadi Y, Andriantoro H, Boom CE, Harimurti K, Romdoni R, et al. Early insertion of intra-aortic balloon pump after cardiac arrest on acute coronary syndrome patients: A Randomized Clinical Trial. Cardiology and Cardiovascular Medicine. 2019;**3**:193-203

[67] Patel NJ, Patel N, Bhardwaj B, Golwala H, Kumar V, Atti V, et al. Trends in utilization of mechanical circulatory support in patients hospitalized after out-of-hospital cardiac arrest. Resuscitation. 2018;**127**:105-113

[68] Bougouin W, Dumas F, Lamhaut L, Marijon E, Carli P, Combes A, et al. Sudden death expertise center investigators. extracorporeal

cardiopulmonary resuscitation in out-of-hospital cardiac arrest: A registry study. European Heart Journal. 2020;**41**(21):1961-1971

[69] Sun T, Guy A, Sidhu A, Finlayson G, Grunau B, Ding L, et al. Veno-arterial extracorporeal membrane oxygenation (VA-ECMO) for emergency cardiac support. Journal of Critical Care. 2018;**44**:31-38

[70] Wang GN, Chen XF, Qiao L, Mei Y, Lv JR, Huang XH, et al. Comparison of extracorporeal and conventional cardiopulmonary resuscitation: A meta-analysis of 2 260 patients with cardiac arrest. World Journal of Emergency Medicine. 2017;**8**(1):5-11

[71] Marinacci LX, Mihatov N, D'Alessandro DA, Villavicencio MA, Roy N, Raz Y, et al. Extracorporeal cardiopulmonary resuscitation (ECPR) survival: A quaternary center analysis. Journal of Cardiac Surgery. 2021;**36**(7):2300-2307

[72] Ryan J. Extracorporeal membrane oxygenation for pediatric cardiac arrest. Critical Care Nurse. 2015;**35**(1):60-69

[73] Huang SC, Wu ET, Wang CC, Chen YS, Chang CI, Chiu IS, et al. Eleven years of experience with extracorporeal cardiopulmonary resuscitation for paediatric patients with in-hospital cardiac arrest. Resuscitation. 2012;**83**(6):710-714

[74] Kalra S, Ranard LS, Memon S, Rao P, Garan AR, Masoumi A, et al. Risk prediction in cardiogenic shock: Current state of knowledge, challenges and opportunities. Journal of Cardiac Failure. 2021;**27**(10):1099-1110

[75] Zweck E, Thayer KL, Helgestad OKL, Kanwar M, Ayouty M, Garan AR, et al. Phenotyping cardiogenic shock. Journal of the American Heart Association. 2021;**10**(14):e020085

[76] Shah M, Patnaik S, Patel B, Ram P, Garg L, Agarwal M, et al. Trends in mechanical circulatory support use and hospital mortality among patients with acute myocardial infarction and non-infarction related cardiogenic shock in the United States. Clinical Research in Cardiology. 2018;**107**(4):287-303

[77] Telukuntla KS, Estep JD. Acute mechanical circulatory support for cardiogenic shock. Methodist DeBakey Cardiovascular Journal. 2020;**16**(1):27-35

[78] Ouyang D, Gulati G, Ha R, Banerjee D. Incidence of temporary mechanical circulatory support before heart transplantation and impact on post-transplant outcomes. The Journal of Heart and Lung Transplantation. 2018;**37**(9):1060-1066

[79] Janssens U, Graf J. Was ist "Schock"? [Shock—What are the basics?]. Internist (Berl). 2004;**45**(3):258-266

[80] Houston MC. Pathophysiology of shock. Critical Care Nursing Clinics of North America. 1990;**2**(2):143-149

[81] Yip HK, Wu CJ, Chang HW, Chen MC, Hang CL, Fang CY, et al. Comparison of impact of primary percutaneous transluminal coronary angioplasty and primary stenting on short-term mortality in patients with cardiogenic shock and evaluation of prognostic. Jpn Heart J. Sep 2002;**43**(5):463-474

[82] Goldberg RJ, Gore JM, Thompson CA, Gurwitz JH. Recent magnitude of and temporal trends (1994-1997) in the incidence and hospital death rates of cardiogenic shock complicating acute myocardial infarction: The second national registry of myocardial infarction. American Heart Journal. 2001;**141**(1):65-72

[83] Hochman JS, Sleeper LA, Webb JG, Sanborn TA, White HD, Talley JD, et al. Early revascularization in acute myocardial infarction complicated by cardiogenic shock. SHOCK Investigators. Should we emergently revascularize occluded coronaries for cardiogenic shock. The New England Journal of Medicine. 1999;**341**(9):625-634

[84] Berger PB, Holmes DR Jr, Stebbins AL, Bates ER, Califf RM, Topol EJ. Impact of an aggressive invasive catheterization and revascularization strategy on mortality in patients with cardiogenic shock in the Global Utilization of Streptokinase and Tissue Plasminogen Activator for Occluded Coronary Arteries (GUSTO-I) trial. An observational study. Circulation. 1997;**96**(1):122-127

[85] Scholz KH, Maier SKG, Maier LS, Lengenfelder B, Jacobshagen C, Jung J, et al. Impact of treatment delay on mortality in ST-segment elevation myocardial infarction (STEMI) patients presenting with and without haemodynamic instability: Results from the German prospective, multicentre FITT-STEMI trial. European Heart Journal. 2018;**39**(13):1065-1074

[86] Thiele H, Ohman EM, de Waha-Thiele S, Zeymer U, Desch S. Management of cardiogenic shock complicating myocardial infarction: An update 2019. European Heart Journal. 2019;**40**(32):2671-2683

[87] Boyd JC, Cox JL, Hassan A, Lutchmedial S, Yip AM, Légaré JF. Where you live in nova scotia can significantly impact your access to lifesaving cardiac care: Access to invasive care influences survival. The Canadian Journal of Cardiology. 2018;**34**(2):202-208

[88] Lemor A, Ya'qoub L, Basir MB. Mechanical circulatory support in acute myocardial infarction and cardiogenic shock. Interventional Cardiology Clinics. 2021;**10**(2):169-184

[89] Reynolds HR, Hochman JS. Cardiogenic shock: Current concepts and improving outcomes. Circulation. 2008;**117**(5):686-697

[90] Zehetgruber M, Mundigler G, Christ G, Merhaut C, Klaar U, Kratochwill C, et al. Relation of hemodynamic variables to augmentation of left anterior descending coronary flow by intraaortic balloon pulsation in coronary artery disease. The American Journal of Cardiology. 1997;**80**(7):951-955

[91] Kimura A, Toyota E, Lu S, Goto M, Yada T, Chiba Y, et al. Effects of intraaortic balloon pumping on septal arterial blood flow velocity waveform during severe left main coronary artery stenosis. Journal of the American College of Cardiology. 1996;**27**(4):810-816

[92] Hochman JS, Buller CE, Sleeper LA, Boland J, Dzavik V, Sanborn TA, et al. Cardiogenic shock complicating acute myocardial infarction—Etiologies, management and outcome: A report from the SHOCK Trial Registry. SHould we emergently revascularize Occluded Coronaries for cardiogenic shocK? Journal of the American College of Cardiology. 2000;**36**(3):1063-1070

[93] Thiele H, Zeymer U, Neumann FJ, Ferenc M, Olbrich HG, Hausleiter J, et al. Intraaortic balloon support for myocardial infarction with cardiogenic shock. The New England Journal of Medicine. 2012;**367**(14):1287-1296

[94] Thiele H, Zeymer U, Neumann FJ, Ferenc M, Olbrich HG, Hausleiter J, et al. Intraaortic Balloon Pump in cardiogenic shock II (IABP-SHOCK II) trial investigators. Intra-aortic balloon

counterpulsation in acute myocardial infarction complicated by cardiogenic shock (IABP-SHOCK II): Final 12 month results of a randomised, open-label trial. Lancet. 2013;**382**(9905):1638-1645

[95] Thiele H, Zeymer U, Thelemann N, Neumann FJ, Hausleiter J, Abdel-Wahab M, et al. Intraaortic balloon pump in cardiogenic shock complicating acute myocardial infarction: Long-term 6-year outcome of the randomized IABP-SHOCK II trial. Circulation. 2019;**139**(3):395-403

[96] Authors/Task Force Members, Windecker S, Kolh P, Alfonso F, Collet JP, Cremer J, et al. 2014 ESC/EACTS Guidelines on myocardial revascularization: The Task Force on Myocardial Revascularization of the European Society of Cardiology (ESC) and the European Association for Cardio-Thoracic Surgery (EACTS)Developed with the special contribution of the European Association of Percutaneous Cardiovascular Interventions (EAPCI). European Heart Journal. 2014;**35**(37):2541-2619

[97] O'Gara PT, Kushner FG, Ascheim DD, Casey DE, Chung MK, de Lemos JA, et al. 2013 ACCF/AHA guideline for the management of ST-elevation myocardial infarction: Executive summary: A report of the American College of Cardiology Foundation/American Heart Association Task Force on Practice Guidelines. Circulation. 2013;**127**(4):529-555

[98] Sheu JJ, Tsai TH, Lee FY, Fang HY, Sun CK, Leu S, et al. Early extracorporeal membrane oxygenator-assisted primary percutaneous coronary intervention improved 30-day clinical outcomes in patients with ST-segment elevation myocardial infarction complicated with profound cardiogenic shock. Critical Care Medicine. 2010;**38**(9):1810-1817

[99] Tsao NW, Shih CM, Yeh JS, Kao YT, Hsieh MH, Ou KL, et al. Extracorporeal membrane oxygenation-assisted primary percutaneous coronary intervention may improve survival of patients with acute myocardial infarction complicated by profound cardiogenic shock. Journal of Critical Care. 2012;**27**(5):530.e1-530.11

[100] Esper SA, Bermudez C, Dueweke EJ, Kormos R, Subramaniam K, Mulukutla S, et al. Extracorporeal membrane oxygenation support in acute coronary syndromes complicated by cardiogenic shock. Catheterization and Cardiovascular Interventions. 2015;**86**(Suppl. 1):S45-S50

[101] Negi SI, Sokolovic M, Koifman E, Kiramijyan S, Torguson R, Lindsay J, et al. Contemporary use of veno-arterial extracorporeal membrane oxygenation for refractory cardiogenic shock in acute coronary syndrome. The Journal of Invasive Cardiology. 2016;**28**(2):52-57

[102] Vallabhajosyula S, Prasad A, Bell MR, Sandhu GS, Eleid MF, Dunlay SM, et al. Extracorporeal membrane oxygenation use in acute myocardial infarction in the United States, 2000 to 2014. Circulation. Heart Failure. 2019;**12**(12):e005929

[103] Zavalichi MA, Nistor I, Nedelcu AE, Zavalichi SD, Georgescu CMA, Stătescu C, et al. Extracorporeal membrane oxygenation in cardiogenic shock due to acute myocardial infarction: A systematic review. BioMed Research International. 2020;**2020**:6126534

[104] Gershlick A. EURO SHOCK testing the value of novel strategy and its cost efficacy in order to improve the poor outcomes in cardiogenic shock. ClinicalTrials.gov identifier: NCT03813134

[105] Thiele H. Prospective randomized multicenter study comparing

extracorporeal life support plus optimal medical care versus optimal medical care alone in patients with acute myocardial infarction complicated by cardiogenic shock undergoing revascularization. ClinicalTrials.gov identifier: NCT03637205

[106] Tsuneyoshi H, Rao V. The role of extracorporeal membrane oxygenation (ECMO) therapy in acute heart failure. International Anesthesiology Clinics. 2012;**50**(3):114-122

[107] Yu K, Long C, Hei F, Li J, Liu J, Ji B, et al. Clinical evaluation of two different extracorporeal membrane oxygenation systems: A single center report. Artificial Organs. 2011;**35**(7):733-737

[108] Lorusso R, Centofanti P, Gelsomino S, Barili F, Di Mauro M, Orlando P, et al. Venoarterial extracorporeal membrane oxygenation for acute fulminant myocarditis in adult patients: A 5-year multi-institutional experience. The Annals of Thoracic Surgery. 2016;**101**(3):919-926

[109] Marasco SF, Vale M, Pellegrino V, Preovolos A, Leet A, Kras A, et al. Extracorporeal membrane oxygenation in primary graft failure after heart transplantation. The Annals of Thoracic Surgery. 2010;**90**(5):1541-1546

[110] Dangers L, Bréchot N, Schmidt M, Lebreton G, Hékimian G, Nieszkowska A, et al. Extracorporeal membrane oxygenation for acute decompensated heart failure. Critical Care Medicine. 2017;**45**(8):1359-1366

[111] Ponikowski P, Voors AA, Anker SD, Bueno H, Cleland JGF, Coats AJS, et al. 2016 ESC Guidelines for the diagnosis and treatment of acute and chronic heart failure: The Task Force for the diagnosis and treatment of acute and chronic heart failure of the European Society of Cardiology (ESC)Developed with the special contribution of the Heart Failure Association (HFA) of the ESC. European Heart Journal. 2016;**37**(27):2129-2200

[112] Sakamoto S, Taniguchi N, Nakajima S, Takahashi A. Extracorporeal life support for cardiogenic shock or cardiac arrest due to acute coronary syndrome. The Annals of Thoracic Surgery. 2012;**94**(1):1-7

[113] Wang SS, Ko WJ, Chen YS, Hsu RB, Chou NK, Chu SH. Mechanical bridge with extracorporeal membrane oxygenation and ventricular assist device to heart transplantation. Artificial Organs. 2001;**25**(8):599-602

[114] Cheng R, Ramzy D, Azarbal B, Arabia FA, Esmailian F, Czer LS, et al. Device strategies for patients in INTERMACS Profiles 1 and 2 cardiogenic shock: Double bridge with extracorporeal membrane oxygenation and initial implant of more durable devices. Artificial Organs. 2017;**41**(3):224-232

[115] Lamhaut L, Jouffroy R, Soldan M, Phillipe P, Deluze T, Jaffry M, et al. Safety and feasibility of prehospital extra corporeal life support implementation by non-surgeons for out-of-hospital refractory cardiac arrest. Resuscitation. 2013;**84**(11):1525-1529

[116] Chakaramakkil MJ, Sivathasan C. ECMO and short-term support for cardiogenic shock in heart failure. Current Cardiology Reports. 2018; **20**(10):87

[117] Lala A, Guo Y, Xu J, Esposito M, Morine K, Karas R, et al. Right ventricular dysfunction in acute myocardial infarction complicated by cardiogenic shock: A Hemodynamic analysis of the should we emergently revascularize occluded coronaries for cardiogenic shock (SHOCK) trial and

registry. Journal of Cardiac Failure. 2018;**24**(3):148-156

[118] Ouweneel DM, Schotborgh JV, Limpens J, Sjauw KD, Engström AE, Lagrand WK, et al. Extracorporeal life support during cardiac arrest and cardiogenic shock: A systematic review and meta-analysis. Intensive Care Medicine. 2016;**42**(12):1922-1934

[119] Burkhoff D, Sayer G, Doshi D, Uriel N. Hemodynamics of mechanical circulatory support. Journal of the American College of Cardiology. 2015;**66**(23):2663-2674

[120] Aubron C, DePuydt J, Belon F, Bailey M, Schmidt M, Sheldrake J, et al. Predictive factors of bleeding events in adults undergoing extracorporeal membrane oxygenation. Annals of Intensive Care. 2016;**6**(1):97

[121] Takayama H, Landes E, Truby L, Fujita K, Kirtane AJ, Mongero L, et al. Feasibility of smaller arterial cannulas in venoarterial extracorporeal membrane oxygenation. The Journal of Thoracic and Cardiovascular Surgery. 2015;**149**(5):1428-1433

[122] Juo YY, Skancke M, Sanaiha Y, Mantha A, Jimenez JC, Benharash P. Efficacy of distal perfusion cannulae in preventing limb ischemia during extracorporeal membrane oxygenation: A systematic review and meta-analysis. Artificial Organs. 2017;**41**(11):E263-E273

[123] Fletcher-Sandersjöö A, Bartek J Jr, Thelin EP, Eriksson A, Elmi-Terander A, Broman M, et al. Predictors of intracranial hemorrhage in adult patients on extracorporeal membrane oxygenation: An observational cohort study. Journal of Intensive Care. 2017;**5**:27

[124] Kasirajan V, Smedira NG, McCarthy JF, Casselman F, Boparai N, McCarthy PM. Risk factors for intracranial hemorrhage in adults on extracorporeal membrane oxygenation. European Journal of Cardio-Thoracic Surgery. 1999;**15**(4):508-514

[125] Gyawali B, Ramakrishna K, Dhamoon AS. Sepsis: The evolution in definition, pathophysiology, and management. SAGE Open Medicine. 2019;**7**:2050

[126] Flierl MA, Rittirsch D, Huber-Lang MS, Sarma JV, Ward PA. Molecular events in the cardiomyopathy of sepsis. Molecular Medicine. 2008;**14**(5-6):327-336

[127] Tsolaki V, Makris D, Mantzarlis K, Zakynthinos E. Sepsis-induced cardiomyopathy: Oxidative implications in the initiation and resolution of the damage. Oxidative Medicine and Cellular Longevity. 2017;**2017**:7393525

[128] Rudiger A, Singer M. Mechanisms of sepsis-induced cardiac dysfunction. Critical Care Medicine. 2007;**35**(6):1599-1608

[129] Chockalingam A, Mehra A, Dorairajan S, Dellsperger KC. Acute left ventricular dysfunction in the critically ill. Chest. 2010;**138**(1):198-207

[130] Dellinger RP, Carlet JM, Masur H, Gerlach H, Calandra T, Cohen J, et al. Surviving Sepsis Campaign guidelines for management of severe sepsis and septic shock. Critical Care Medicine. 2004;**32**(3):858-873

[131] Bartlett RH, Roloff DW, Custer JR, Younger JG, Hirschl RB. Extracorporeal life support: The University of Michigan experience. Journal of the American Medical Association. 2000;**283**(7):904-908

[132] Butt WW, Chiletti R. ECMO for neonatal sepsis in 2019. Frontiers in Pediatrics. 2020;**8**:50

[133] Bartlett RH. Extracorporeal support for septic shock. Pediatric Critical Care Medicine. 2007;**8**(5):498-499

[134] Bruni FD, Komwatana P, Soulsby ME, Hess ML. Endotoxin and myocardial failure: Role of the myofibril and venous return. The American Journal of Physiology. 1978;**235**(2):H150-H156

[135] Cunnion RE, Schaer GL, Parker MM, Natanson C, Parrillo JE. The coronary circulation in human septic shock. Circulation. 1986;**73**(4):637-644

[136] Flesch M, Kilter H, Cremers B, Laufs U, Südkamp M, Ortmann M, et al. Effects of endotoxin on human myocardial contractility involvement of nitric oxide and peroxynitrite. Journal of the American College of Cardiology. 1999;**33**(4):1062-1070

[137] Natanson C, Eichenholz PW, Danner RL, Eichacker PQ, Hoffman WD, Kuo GC, et al. Endotoxin and tumor necrosis factor challenges in dogs simulate the cardiovascular profile of human septic shock. The Journal of Experimental Medicine. 1989;**169**(3):823-832

[138] Kumar A, Thota V, Dee L, Olson J, Uretz E, Parrillo JE. Tumor necrosis factor alpha and interleukin 1beta are responsible for in vitro myocardial cell depression induced by human septic shock serum. The Journal of Experimental Medicine. 1996;**183**(3):949-958

[139] Shah AM, Spurgeon HA, Sollott SJ, Talo A, Lakatta EG. 8-bromo-cGMP reduces the myofilament response to Ca2+ in intact cardiac myocytes. Circulation Research. 1994;**74**(5):970-978

[140] Habimana R, Choi I, Cho HJ, Kim D, Lee K, Jeong I. Sepsis-induced cardiac dysfunction: A review of pathophysiology. Acute Critical Care. 2020;**35**(2):57-66

[141] Crouser ED, Julian MW, Blaho DV, Pfeiffer DR. Endotoxin-induced mitochondrial damage correlates with impaired respiratory activity. Critical Care Medicine. 2002;**30**(2):276-284

[142] Brealey D, Brand M, Hargreaves I, Heales S, Land J, Smolenski R, et al. Association between mitochondrial dysfunction and severity and outcome of septic shock. Lancet. 2002;**360**(9328):219-223

[143] Crouser ED, Julian MW, Huff JE, Joshi MS, Bauer JA, Gadd ME, et al. Abnormal permeability of inner and outer mitochondrial membranes contributes independently to mitochondrial dysfunction in the liver during acute endotoxemia. Critical Care Medicine. 2004;**32**(2):478-488

[144] Larche J, Lancel S, Hassoun SM, Favory R, Decoster B, Marchetti P, et al. Inhibition of mitochondrial permeability transition prevents sepsis-induced myocardial dysfunction and mortality. Journal of the American College of Cardiology. 2006;**48**(2):377-385

[145] Kirov MY, Evgenov OV, Evgenov NV, Egorina EM, Sovershaev MA, Sveinbjørnsson B, et al. Infusion of methylene blue in human septic shock: A pilot, randomized, controlled study. Critical Care Medicine. 2001;**29**(10):1860-1867

[146] Forfia PR, Watkins SP, Rame JE, Stewart KJ, Shapiro EP. Relationship between B-type natriuretic peptides and pulmonary capillary wedge pressure in the intensive care unit. Journal of the American College of Cardiology. 2005;**45**(10):1667-1671

[147] Jefic D, Lee JW, Jefic D, Savoy-Moore RT, Rosman HS. Utility

of B-type natriuretic peptide and N-terminal pro B-type natriuretic peptide in evaluation of respiratory failure in critically ill patients. Chest. 2005;**128**(1):288-295

[148] Røsjø H, Varpula M, Hagve TA, Karlsson S, Ruokonen E, Pettilä V, et al. Circulating high sensitivity troponin T in severe sepsis and septic shock: Distribution, associated factors, and relation to outcome. Intensive Care Medicine. 2011;**37**(1):77-85

[149] Repessé X, Charron C, Vieillard-Baron A. Evaluation of left ventricular systolic function revisited in septic shock. Critical Care. 2013;**17**(4):164

[150] Vallabhajosyula S, Kumar M, Pandompatam G, Sakhuja A, Kashyap R, Kashani K, et al. Prognostic impact of isolated right ventricular dysfunction in sepsis and septic shock: An 8-year historical cohort study. Annals of Intensive Care. 2017;**7**(1):94

[151] Landesberg G, Gilon D, Meroz Y, Georgieva M, Levin PD, Goodman S, et al. Diastolic dysfunction and mortality in severe sepsis and septic shock. European Heart Journal. 2012;**33**(7):895-903

[152] Ng PY, Sin WC, Ng AK, Chan WM. Speckle tracking echocardiography in patients with septic shock: A case control study (SPECKSS). Critical Care. 2016;**20**(1):145

[153] Falk L, Hultman J, Broman LM. Extracorporeal membrane oxygenation for septic shock. Critical Care Medicine. 2019;**47**(8):1097-1105

[154] Bréchot N, Luyt CE, Schmidt M, Leprince P, Trouillet JL, Léger P, et al. Venoarterial extracorporeal membrane oxygenation support for refractory cardiovascular dysfunction during severe bacterial septic shock. Critical Care Medicine. 2013;**41**(7):1616-1626

[155] Bréchot N, Hajage D, Kimmoun A, Demiselle J, Agerstrand C, Montero S, et al. Venoarterial extracorporeal membrane oxygenation to rescue sepsis-induced cardiogenic shock: A retrospective, multicentre, international cohort study. Lancet. 2020;**396**(10250):545-552

[156] Jardin F, Brun-Ney D, Auvert B, Beauchet A, Bourdarias JP. Sepsis-related cardiogenic shock. Critical Care Medicine. 1990;**18**(10):1055-1060

[157] Vogel DJ, Murray J, Czapran AZ, Camporota L, Ioannou N, Meadows CIS, et al. Veno-arterio-venous ECMO for septic cardiomyopathy: A single-centre experience. Perfusion. 2018;**33**(1):57-64

[158] Sangli SS, Noronha SF, Mourad B, Jean R, Bohman JK, Seelhammer TG. A systematic review of preexisting sepsis and extracorporeal membrane oxygenation. ASAIO Journal. 2020;**66**(1):1-7

[159] Maclaren G, Butt W. Extracorporeal membrane oxygenation and sepsis. Critical Care and Resuscitation. 2007;**9**(1):76-80

[160] Riera J, Romay E, Ferrer R. Management of myocardial dysfunction in septic shock. Potential role of extracorporeal membrane oxygenation. Medical Intensiva (Engl Ed). 2018;**42**(5):301-305

[161] Ling RR, Ramanathan K, Poon WH, Tan CS, Brechot N, Brodie D, et al. Venoarterial extracorporeal membrane oxygenation as mechanical circulatory support in adult septic shock: A systematic review and meta-analysis with individual participant data meta-regression analysis. Critical Care. 2021;**25**(1):246

[162] Nabzdyk CS, Couture EJ, Shelton K, Cudemus G, Bittner EA. Sepsis induced cardiomyopathy: Pathophysiology and use of mechanical circulatory support for refractory shock. Journal of Critical Care. 2019;**54**:228-234

[163] Esper SA, Levy JH, Waters JH, Welsby IJ. Extracorporeal membrane oxygenation in the adult: A review of anticoagulation monitoring and transfusion. Anesthesia and Analgesia. 2014;**118**(4):731-743

[164] Tonna JE, Abrams D, Brodie D, Greenwood JC, Rubio Mateo-Sidron JA, Usman A, et al. Management of adult patients supported with venovenous extracorporeal membrane oxygenation (VV ECMO): Guideline from the Extracorporeal Life Support Organization (ELSO). ASAIO Journal. 2021;**67**(6):601-610

[165] Brogan TV, Lequier L, Lorusso R, MacLaren G, Peek G. Extracorporeal Life Support: The ELSO Red Book. (5th ed.) ed. Extracorporeal Life Support Organization; 2017

[166] Lorusso R, Shekar K, MacLaren G, Schmidt M, Pellegrino V, Meyns B, et al. ELSO Interim guidelines for venoarterial extracorporeal membrane oxygenation in adult cardiac patients. ASAIO Journal. 2021;**67**(8):827-844

[167] Seelhammer TG, Bohman JK, Schulte PJ, Hanson AC, Aganga DO. Comparison of bivalirudin versus heparin for maintenance systemic anticoagulation during adult and pediatric extracorporeal membrane oxygenation. Critical Care Medicine. 2021;**49**(9):1481-1492

[168] Ortoleva J, Roberts RJ, Devine LT, French A, Kawabori M, Chen F, et al. Methylene Blue for vasoplegia during extracorporeal membrane oxygenation support. Journal of Cardiothoracic and Vascular Anesthesia. 2021;**35**(9):2694-2699

[169] Porizka M, Rulisek J, Flaksa M, Otahal M, Lips M, Belohlavek J, et al. Dual veno-arterial extra-corporeal membrane oxygenation support in a patient with refractory hyperdynamic septic shock: A case report. Perfusion. 2022;**37**(3):306-310

[170] Scherer M, Sirat AS, Moritz A, Martens S. Extracorporeal membrane oxygenation as perioperative right ventricular support in patients with biventricular failure undergoing left ventricular assist device implantation. European Journal of Cardio-Thoracic Surgery. 2011;**39**(6):939-944

[171] Bonicolini E, Martucci G, Simons J, Raffa GM, Spina C, Lo Coco V, et al. Limb ischemia in peripheral veno-arterial extracorporeal membrane oxygenation: A narrative review of incidence, prevention, monitoring, and treatment. Critical Care. 2019;**23**(1):266

[172] Lindholm JA. Cannulation for veno-venous extracorporeal membrane oxygenation. Journal of Thoracic Disease. 2018;**10**(Suppl. 5):S606-S612

[173] Kimmoun A, Oulehri W, Sonneville R, Grisot PH, Zogheib E, Amour J, et al. Prevalence and outcome of heparin-induced thrombocytopenia diagnosed under veno-arterial extracorporeal membrane oxygenation: A retrospective nationwide study. Intensive Care Medicine. 2018;**44**(9):1460-1469